AMERICAN MIDWIVES

AMERICAN MIDWIVES

1860 to the Present

Judy Barrett Litoff

Contributions in Medical History, Number 1

GREENWOOD PRESS
Westport, Connecticut • London, England

Library of Congress Cataloging in Publication Data

Litoff, Judy Barrett.
   American midwives, 1860 to the present.

   (Contributions in medical history ; no. 1 ISSN 0147-1058)
   An outgrowth of the author's thesis, University of Maine at Orono.
   Bibliography: p.
   1. Midwives—United States—History. I. Title. II. Series: Contributions in medical
history ; no. 1.
   RG960.L58   618.2   77-83893
   ISBN 0-8371-9824-0

Library of Congress Catalog Card Number: 77-83893
ISBN: 0-8371-9824-0
ISSN: 0147-1058

First published in 1978

Greenwood Press, Inc.
51 Riverside Avenue, Westport, Connecticut 06880

Printed in the United States of America

10 9 8 7 6 5 4 3 2 1

For Nadja and Alyssa

Contents

Preface

I first considered undertaking a historical study of American midwives after reading Frances E. Kobrin's "The American Midwife Controversy: A Crisis of Professionalization" (*Bulletin of the History of Medicine*, 40 [July-August, 1966], 350-363). At the time, fall 1971, I was just beginning my doctoral studies in history at the University of Maine at Orono. The circumstances surrounding the birth of my daughter, Nadja, in May 1972, who was delivered by an obstetrician in a hospital, made me even more curious about the history of the American midwife and the forces which brought about her near elimination. I discovered that researchers had neglected the midwife's history, even though as late as 1910 she attended one-half of all births in the United States. My interest in midwives, coupled with a larger commitment to uncovering woman's past, convinced me that the changing role of the midwife in American society between 1860 and the present would make an appropriate study.

A brief note clarifying the use of the terms *midwifery* and *obstetrics* is in order. Prior to the midwife debate of the early years of the twentieth century, the two terms were used synonymously. Professors of midwifery were appointed to the faculties of medical schools, and textbooks on midwifery for medical students and practitioners were published. It was not until the second and third decades of the twentieth century that Americans began to make distinctions between the two terms, with *midwifery* referring to the practices of midwives and *obstetrics* to the work of highly trained physicians. Even today, however, the two terms are similarly defined in standard American medical dictionaries. Nevertheless, popular usage has caused the two terms to be distinguished from each other. In this work, I have used *midwifery* and *obstetrics* synonymously when discussing the period prior to 1900. For the post-1900 era, the different interpretations of the two terms have been employed.[1]

The definitive history of American midwives since 1860 is yet to be written. For example, a great deal of information concerning legal proscriptions and regulations, training and regulatory programs, and the attitudes of public health officials toward early twentieth-century midwives can be gleaned by examining the records of the various state boards of health for the 1900-1930 period. Undoubtedly, individual state studies will bring to light additional statistical information regarding the complicated and controversial question of the number and percentage of infant and maternal deaths for which midwives were responsible. For this study, however, I examined the records of only six states (Connecticut, Georgia, Maine, Massachusetts, New Jersey, and Rhode Island) and one city (New York). Uneven amounts of information on ten other states was also gathered. Because of the dearth of published information on the subject, I felt it was appropriate to continue with this work.

Numerous individuals went out of their way to make this book possible. Janet Hogan, Director of the Interlibrary Loan Division of the Raymond H. Fogler Library at the University of Maine at Orono, made sure that I quickly received my numerous interlibrary loan requests. Without her assistance, this study would have never materialized. Similarly, Melda W. Page, chief librarian at the Veterans Administration Center in Togus, Maine, aided me in my search for materials not available in the immediate area. Dorothy Wertz and Richard Wertz allowed me to read their unpublished manuscript, "Lying-in, A History of Childbirth in America: Its Technologies and Social Relations" (Boston, [1974]). The support and encouragement I received from my dissertation advisor, Professor David C. Smith, were invaluable. Finally, a very special thanks is due to two people who have helped me in an untold number of ways—Dorothy Wooddall Barrett and Hal Litoff.

NOTES

1. Joseph B. De Lee, "Obstetrics vs. Midwifery," *Journal of the American Medical Association,* 103 (August 1934), 307; Josiah Morris Slemons, "Progress in Obstetrics: 1890-1940," *American Journal of Surgery,* 51 (1941), 80. A few of the late nineteenth-century midwifery texts for medical students and practitioners include the following: Alfred L. Galabin, *A Manual of Midwifery* (Philadelphia, 1886); Henry J. Garrigues, *Practical Guide in Antiseptic Midwifery in Hospitals and Private Practice* (Detroit, 1886); Rodney Glisan, *Textbook of Modern Midwifery* (Philadelphia, 1881). Thomas L. Stedman, *Stedman's Medical Dictionary,* 22nd ed. (Baltimore, 1972).

AMERICAN MIDWIVES

1

The Midwife Throughout History: A Brief Overview to 1860

Midwifery has been the almost exclusive province of women throughout recorded history. Indeed, considerable evidence exists which indicates that the management of labor has traditionally been considered the responsibility of women. Several references to the work of midwives can be found in the Bible. Exodus 1:15-22 relates the experiences of two Hebrew midwives, Shiphrah and Puah, who refused to follow the Egyptian king's command requiring that they kill all infant males. When the midwives were questioned by the king for failing to follow his order, they replied: ". . . Hebrew women are not like the Egyptian women; for they are vigorous and are delivered before the midwife comes to them." This passage indicates that the presence of a midwife was considered sufficient when an attendant at birth was necessary and that parturition was believed to be such a normal process that many births went unattended.[1] The writings of classical Greek and Roman physicians, such as Hippocrates, Galen, and Celsus, provide further information about the regularity with which the midwife served as the attendant at birth. These writers supply evidence that male physicians were summoned only when special emergencies or difficulties arose.[2]

Throughout the Middle Ages, the midwife continued to serve as the attendant at birth for rich and poor alike. The significant role played by the midwife in England at this time can be illustrated by the fact that in 1554 the Church began administering an oath requiring that she be "diligent and faithful and ready to help every woman labouring with child as well as the poor as the rich. . . ." The oath prohibited the midwife from exercising witchcraft or using charms, invocations, or prayers not allowed by the Church, and it warned against the presence of men in the lying-in chamber except in extreme emergencies.[3] The Church also allowed and encouraged midwives to perform infant baptism when a priest was not available.[4]

Midwives also played a central role in the birth process in colonial America. One of the earliest midwives in the Massachusetts Bay Colony was Bridget Lee Fuller, wife of Deacon Samuel Fuller. She traveled on the *Mayflower* and probably aided in the three births that occurred during the Atlantic crossing. She continued to serve as a midwife at Plymouth until her death in 1664.[5] Epitaphs of various other women further attest to their value as midwives. The inscription on the tombstone of Ann Eliot, the wife of the Indian missionary, John Eliot, bears testimony to her services as a midwife.[6] The epitaph of Elizabeth Phillips, whose death in 1761 brought an end to her more than forty-year career as a New England midwife, stated that she had "by ye blessing of God, . . .brought into this world above three thousand children."[7] Perhaps the most famous midwife of the colonial period was Anne Hutchinson. Although she is most remembered for her leading role in the Antinomian controversy of the 1630s, she was also "very helpful in the times of childbirth, and other occasions of bodily infirmities and well furnished with means for those purposes."[8]

It was the practice of the colony of New Amsterdam to appoint an official Town Midwife. In 1660, New Amsterdam allotted this official a salary of 100 guilders per year for attending the poor. In the southern colonies it was not unusual for each plantation to have its own midwife. Often, she would be a slave who served both white and black women. White women also acted as midwives and frequently were paid in kind as was the case of the midwife, Thorpe, of Surrey County, Virginia, who in 1685 charged a fee of 100 pounds of tobacco for her services.[9]

Most colonial midwives were held in high esteem by the community. Those women who were unfortunate enough to be present at the birth of deformed or stillborn infants, however, were sometimes suspected of practicing witchcraft. Jane Hawkins, a well-known midwife and friend of Anne Hutchinson, delivered the still-born "monstrosity" of Mary Dyer. This birth was the subject of much debate and speculation among New Englanders, and John Winthrop denounced Hawkins as "notorious for familiarity with the devil." So much discussion followed concerning the possibility of Hawkins's being a witch that in 1638 the magistrates prohibited her from practicing medicine.[10]

Few rules and regulations regarding the practices of midwives existed in colonial America. This is not surprising in light of the fact that all medical practitioners—physicians, surgeons, and midwives—were allowed to pursue their careers with little supervision until the second half of the eighteenth century. Moreover, birth was viewed as a natural process in which a minimal amount of specialized knowledge was required.[11] Consequently, any woman who had borne children and had assisted with the births of a few family members or friends could rightfully be designated a midwife.

At least one colony did attempt to regulate the practices of midwives during the early eighteenth century. In 1716, the New York Common Council enacted a law, modeled after the 1554 English oath, which required that the midwife "be diligent and ready to help any woman in labor, whether poor or rich. . . ." It included no provisions for the examination of the midwife's skills, and it made no mention of the presence of men in the lying-in chamber. In the 1730s, the law was amended to require that the midwife not "open any mystery apertaining to . . . [her] Office, in the presence of any Man unless Necessity . . ." so demanded.[12]

New York was not the only colony which endeavored to keep men out of the lying-in chamber. As early as 1646, a man in Maine was prosecuted for acting as a midwife.[13] Generally, neither male physicians nor husbands were welcomed in the lying-in chamber, and midwives held a virtual monopoly in this field. It was not considered improper, however, for midwives to turn to physicians for assistance when certain emergencies arose. If version was necessary, for instance, the aid of a physician was usually required.[14] Midwives did not use forceps nor did they have the instruments necessary to perform embryulcia.[15] Doctors were also summoned on those rare occasions when cesarean operations were performed.

Very few records of colonial and early national midwives have survived to the present. No eyewitness account of childbirth during the colonial period is known to exist.[16] Journals and diaries of midwives are also difficult to locate. Susanna Müller of Providence Township, Lancaster County, Pennsylvania, kept a record of her experiences as a midwife for the years 1791-1815. Unfortunately, her memoirs have not been published. The diary of Martha Moore Ballard, a midwife in Augusta, Maine, and the surrounding towns during the late eighteenth and early nineteenth centuries, is somewhat easier to obtain. Ballard's work, which covers the years 1785-1812 and is more than 200 pages in length, has been reprinted. It provides important information about the day-to-day activities of the midwife of the late eighteenth century.[17]

Due to the paucity of primary sources, it is difficult to make an accurate assessment about the state of knowledge of the average colonial midwife.[18] In most instances, she provided moral support and encouragement to the parturient woman and, otherwise, let nature take its course. Mild herbal remedies for pain were sometimes employed, but midwives did not make use of bloodletting, purging, or other "heroic" medical practices. At this time, there was little knowledge of either antisepsis or asepsis, and thus, no special precautions concerning cleanliness were undertaken. Many midwives carried collapsible birthstools in their bags, but not every parturient woman used the sitting posture. Variations of the supine position were also practiced. Formal instruction for American midwives did not exist until the 1760s, and firsthand experience and observation furnished the best training program for the prospective midwife.

Some midwifery manuals were in circulation, although it is impossible to determine to what extent they were read or how carefully the average midwife followed their instructions. Seventeenth-century midwives who could read might have been familiar with Thomas Raynolde's *Byrth of Mankynde*, the first book in English to deal with the subject of midwifery. It appeared in 1540 and was a translation of a Latin work, Eucharius Rösslin's *Rosengarten* (1514), or *A Rosegarden for Pregnant Women and Midwives*. Included in *Byrth of Mankynde* were references to the birthstool and podalic version. The first book written by an English midwife on midwifery was Jane Sharp's *The Midwives Book, or the Whole Art of Midwifery; Directing Childbearing Women How to Behave* (1671).[19]

Probably another book of interest to midwives in colonial America was a work by the very famous eighteenth-century English midwife, Elizabeth Nihell. In 1760, she published *A Treatise on the Art of Midwifery. Setting Forth Various abuses therein, especially as to the practice with Instruments: the Whole serving to put all Rational Inquirers in a fair way of very safely forming their own Judgment upon the Question; which it is best to employ, In Cases of Pregnancy and Lying-In, a Man-Midwife or, a Midwife.*

Nihell's book was one of the first published works that discussed the propriety of male midwives serving as attendants at births.[20] Prior to the late eighteenth century, the presence of men in the lying-in chamber was so rare that there was little cause for debate or discussion of this subject. No record is even known to exist of a man attending a *normal* birth until 1663. In that year, Louis XIV of France engaged Julien Clement to attend the labor of his mistress, Louise de la Vallière, because he feared that the *sage-femmes* would not be able to keep the birth a secret.[21] The desire for secrecy, however, played a rather inconsequential role in providing a rationale for permitting men to enter the lying-in chamber. Much more important was the gradual development of scientific midwifery.

Probably the single most important event which prepared the way for the acceptance of midwifery as a science, and, as a consequence, brought about the displacement of midwives, was the development of the obstetric forceps by the British surgeon, Peter Chamberlen, the Elder, early in the seventeenth century.[22] For almost 100 years, the Chamberlens kept the forceps a family secret. In order to insure secrecy, the parturient woman was blindfolded, and the forceps were carried into the lying-in chamber in a large wooden box covered with gilded carvings. Gradually, physicians either bought "the secret" from the Chamberlens or developed their own version of the forceps. Midwives could not afford to buy the forceps nor could they find physicians who would instruct them in their proper use.[23]

The research and writings of the British physician William Smellie (1697-1763) played a prominent role in popularizing the forceps and in opening the doors of the lying-in chamber to men. In the 1740s and 1750s, Smellie taught classes in midwifery to more than 900 students. Generally, he demonstrated his procedures on mannequins, but occasionally he delivered poor women in their homes at no charge in return for his classes to observe. By making precise measurements of the female pelvis, Smellie was able to use the forceps without mutilating the newborn infant.[24] At about this same time, the establishment of lying-in hospitals for the poor of London enabled men to make even greater inroads into the lying-in chamber.

Some midwives were quite outspoken in their opposition to having men serve as attendants at birth. Elizabeth Nihell angrily attacked Smellie and vehemently opposed the growth of male midwifery. In her 1760 *Treatise on the Art of Midwifery*, she alluded to Smellie's hand as "the delicate fist of a great horse-godmother of a he midwife." She scoffed at

that multitude of disciples of Dr. Smellie, trained up at the feet of his artificial doll—in short, those self-constituted men midwives made out of broken barbers, tailors, or even pork butchers; for I know myself one of the last trade who, after passing his life in stuffing sausages, is turned an intrepid physician and man midwife.[25]

Despite the protestations of Nihell and her growing number of supporters, the concept of male midwifery was accepted by the English upper classes by the last half of the eighteenth century.[26] Meanwhile, the status of midwives continued to decline because it was generally believed that women were incapable of understanding and performing the obstetric techniques that were being developed.

The advances in obstetric knowledge and the increased acceptance of men in the lying-in chamber in England soon made an impact on midwifery practices in America. Several prominent eighteenth-century American physicians, including William Shippen, Jr., of Philadelphia, received the M.D. degree at the University of Edinburgh and studied in London under disciples of Smellie. Upon returning to America, these physicians put into practice the obstetric knowledge that they had learned in England. Unlike most of his contemporaries, Shippen used the information he had garnered in England to develop a series of pioneering lectures on midwifery which he offered to both men and women beginning in 1765. He explained that he had planned the course in midwifery in order to instruct those women who have virtue enough to own their ignorance and apply for instructions, as well as those young gentlemen now engaged in the study of that useful and necessary branch of surgery who are taking pains to qualify themselves to practice in different parts of the country with safety and advantage to their fellow citizens.[27]

It is impossible to estimate how many women and men Shippen trained, but one medical historian has estimated that as late as 1800, midwives who studied under Shippen were still practicing and that they "probably had as good a course as was then available in this country."[28]

It was not a simple task for American physicians in the colonial period to convince men and women that they were entitled to serve as attendants at birth during ordinary labors.[29] The development of formal medical education in America, however, provided potential male midwives with a decided advantage over their female counterparts. By the end of the eighteenth century, four medical schools, all restricted to male students, had been established on American soil.[30] This meant that women were being systematically excluded from attaining a medical education at the precise time when knowledge of the scientific advances in obstetrics would have enabled them to become more competent midwives. Once this process had begun, it became increasingly difficult for midwives to keep up with the medical discoveries of the nineteenth century which eventually brought about the development of modern obstetrics.

Women interested in midwifery had to resort to training through private sources, or, on occasion, to classes, such as those conducted by William Shippen. In most instances, they were encouraged to attend only normal births. For example, Dr. Valentine Seaman, a midwifery specialist of the post-revolutionary war period, instructed midwives in how to deal with abnormal cases of labor and he even allowed his female students to practice version on a mannequin. Nevertheless, he made it clear that this was "a part of the business, well for you *to know*, but not politic for you to practise."[31] Dr. Samuel Bard, Seaman's contemporary, was also concerned about the education of American midwives. In an attempt to correct some of their errors, he published a *Compendium of the Theory and Practice of Midwifery* in 1807. Because the book was both inexpensive and easy to understand, it was quite successful and by 1819 it had gone through five editions. Bard also opposed the use of instruments by women, and he stressed that the midwife's major responsibility was to let nature take its course.[32]

As the number of men who were trained in obstetrics increased, the number of parturient women who called on physicians for normal deliveries grew as well. The challenge from physicians caused colonial midwives to resort quite frequently to newspaper advertisements in an attempt to attract more patients. Throughout the 1770s and 1780s, midwives and physicians advertised in New York newspapers in the hope of swaying public opinion.[33] Competition in Boston was perhaps even greater than in New York, and one midwife, Mary Bass, announced in 1772 that she was moving from Boston to Salem because "men midwives are fairly numerous in Boston."[34]

Midwives were generally unsuccessful in their campaign against trained physicians, and by the beginning of the nineteenth century male midwifery had become firmly established in America.[35] Admittedly, modesty prevented some parturient women and their husbands from employing physicians. Of equal importance was the fact that high physicians' fees prohibited families with poor and moderate incomes from engaging men. By 1800, however, it was quite fashionable for upper-class women in urban areas to enlist physicians as accoucheurs.

The male-midwifery debate increased in intensity as the number of men in the lying-in chamber grew. During the first half of the nineteenth century numerous books and pamphlets on this topic were published in both the United States and England. Significantly, the most vocal opponents and supporters of male midwifery were physicians.

The principal argument employed by the male-midwifery opponents was that the presence of a man in the lying-in chamber offended the sense of modesty and delicacy of the parturient woman. Thomas Ewell, one of the leading American physicians opposed to male midwifery, insisted that the male accoucheur so greatly offended the woman in the midst of labor that her contractions often completely subsided. Ewell also related the case of a prominent physician who "infuriated with the sight of the woman he had just delivered, leaped into her bed before she was restored to a state of nature." He further maintained that midwives could be trained to handle normal deliveries and that they were capable of conducting vaginal examinations and simple forms of version.[36]

An anonymous pamphlet published in 1851, *An Appeal to the Medical Society of Rhode-Island, in Behalf of Woman to be Restored to her Natural Rights as "Midwife" and Elevated by Education to be the Physician of her Own Sex,* reinforced the views of Ewell. The author argued that there was abundant proof that women could serve with distinction as midwives. "Where, then," asked the writer, "is the excuse for the indecencies and outrages of man-midwifery? Why is it that, without the plea of necessity, our wives are exposed to the shame and pollution of examinations, which are INVARI-ABLE, and manipulations, such as a pure-minded and sensitive woman must blush to think of—such as must excite the indignation of every man who regards the person of his wife as sacred!"[37]

The moral emphasis of the early nineteenth-century male-mid-wifery opponents has caused one historian to conclude that they were "motivated not by a desire to broaden opportunities for women, but by the wish to remove from society the paradox created by conflicting demands of modesty and safety." These opponents, who were primarily men, wanted to keep physicians out of the lying-in chamber "only incidentally to give employment to women." Rather, they supported the midwife in the name of morality and decency. They were not, for the most part, acting in behalf of the women's rights movement of the early nineteenth century.[38]

In an attempt to discredit the work of men in the lying-in chamber, male-midwifery opponents also criticized physicians for resorting too frequently to "iron instruments," a label deridingly applied to the forceps. The author of *An Appeal to the Medical Society of Rhode-Island* argued that "twenty women now die in childbed, and a hundred are tortured with instruments, where there would not be one, if women, only, officiated as midwives; in fact, the very in-struments were never invented or required until the assumption of man as midwife. . . ." Male-midwifery critics also accused physi-cians of turning to "ergot, to stupifying chloroform, the crushing forceps, or the murderous perforator" in order to bring about more prompt deliveries.[39] Thus, the critics repeatedly used the phrase, "meddlesome midwifery" when describing the practices of the physicians. They also charged physicians with taking on normal midwifery cases in order to build up large medical practices. Surprisingly, statements by male-midwifery proponents generally supported this view. In speaking to the students at Albany Medical College, Dr. John Van Pelt Quackenbush urged the prospective doctors to take on as many obstetric cases as possible. "Who holds the key, that opens a large practice to the general practitioner," asked Quackenbush, "if the accoucheur does not?"[40]

During the first half of the nineteenth century, many of the male-midwifery opponents called for the training of midwives. Not until Samuel Gregory established the Boston Female Medical College in 1848 were American midwives able to receive formal schooling. In the mid-1840s, Gregory began both writing and lecturing on the evils of men in the lying-in chamber and on the need to educate women in medicine. By November 1848, he had solicited enough money and support to begin offering a three-month course of instruction in midwifery. Twelve women attended the first course, and between the fall of 1848 and the spring of 1851, six courses in midwifery were offered. During its first three years of existence, the Boston Female Medical College did not offer a program leading to the M.D. degree, but it did award certificates in midwifery upon successful completion of the course. In 1851, the name of the school was changed to the New England Female Medical College, and in February 1852, the course of instruction was expanded to include a full medical education. From 1852 until financial difficulties forced it to merge with the homeopathic medical school at Boston University in 1874, the New England Medical College offered the M.D. degree.[41]

Proponents of male midwifery harshly criticized Gregory and other supporters of the midwife. Members of the Boston Medical Society even intimated that the young bachelor without his M.D. degree had a prurient interest in pregnant women. The editor of the official journal of the Boston Medical Society characterized Gregory's notions as "altogether unchaste, and from their nature, calculated to beget a prurience of thought at once at variance with propriety, and at war with the first principles of virtue."[42]

Another argument used by male-midwifery advocates was that women lacked the ability to become competent birth attendants.

Such remarks were directed not only toward midwives but also toward the growing number of female physicians in the United States, such as Emily Blackwell, Harriot K. Hunt, and Marie Zakrzewska. In an age when domesticity and motherhood were considered the only proper functions of "ladies," young women who desired careers which would take them away from the home faced ridicule from large segments of the population. Moreover, the established nineteenth-century medical view of woman was that she was a frail creature, dominated by her emotions. Women allegedly lacked the intellectual capacity to become midwives or physicians. Many doctors were convinced that the uterus and central nervous system were closely connected. Shocks to the nervous system, such as prolonged or intense study, might, in turn, prohibit a woman's reproductive organs from growing to full maturity. Physicians argued that those women who dared to engage in serious intellectual pursuits, such as the study of medicine, faced the grave risk of being unable to produce normal, healthy children.[43]

In an attempt to bolster their position, male-midwifery proponents also emphasized the potential dangers of pregnancy. They related countless stories of women who had died in childbirth because the midwife had waited too long in summoning the doctor. Critics of male midwifery could not easily overlook these stories since they, too, agreed that physicians should be enlisted during preternatural labors. In fact, virtually everyone assumed that the skills of the physician were necessary during complicated or abnormal births. Consequently, courses in midwifery and the diseases of women and children were included in the curricula of the burgeoning numbers of medical schools established in the United States throughout the nineteenth century. Although not every medical school had a separate chair of midwifery, the inclusion of midwifery in the curricula of medical schools was an indication of the inroads physicians had made in a field that had once been dominated by women.[44]

By the decade of the 1860s, the debate over male midwifery had somewhat subsided. Certainly, the moral issue of whether or not a man's presence in the lying-in chamber was offensive no longer elicited the vehement emotional response that it had during the first half of the nineteenth century. Most late nineteenth-century manuals for mothers and pregnant women were written with the assumption that the parturient woman would hire both a physician and monthly nurse for her confinement.[45] Male physicians no longer found it necessary to battle for the right to enter the lying-in chamber. They had won acceptance as accoucheurs among urban, middle- and upper-class Americans.

NOTES

1. See also Genesis 35:17; 38:28.

2. William Goodell, "When and Why Were Male Physicians Employed as Accoucheurs?" *American Journal of Obstetrics and the Diseases of Women and Children,* 9 (August 1876), 381.

3. Quoted in J. H. Aveling, *English Midwives, Their History and Prospects* (London, 1967; reprint of 1872 edition) pp. 90-93.

4. Many historians contend that it was the question of infant baptism that precipitated the licensing of midwives by the Church of England. See, for example, Harvey Graham, *Eternal Eve: The Mysteries of Birth and the Customs That Surround It* (London, 1960), p. 104.

5. I. Snapper, "Midwifery, Past and Present," *Bulletin of the New York Academy of Medicine,* 39 (August 1963), 503-504.

6. Roy E. Nicodemus, "The History of American Obstetrics," *Centaur,* 51 (1945-1946), 26.

7. Quoted in Francis R. Packard, *History of Medicine in the United States* (New York, 1931), I, 49.

8. Quoted in Herbert Thoms, *Chapters in American Obstetrics* (Springfield, Ill., 1933), p. 10.

9. Snapper, "Midwifery," 506; Nicodemus, "History," 26.

10. John Winthrop, *A Short Story of the Rise, Reign and Ruin of the Antinomians, Familists and Libertines* (1644). Quoted in David D. Hall, ed., *The Antinomian Controversy, 1636-1638* (Middletown, Conn., 1968), p. 281.

11. The belief that birth was a natural process should not be misconstrued as meaning that the colonial population correctly understood the physiology of pregnancy and parturition. Rather, birth was deemed natural in that it was usually regarded in a matter-of-fact manner. See Charles E. Nash, *The History of Augusta: First Settlements and Early Days as A Town, Including the Diary of Mrs. Martha Moore Ballard* (Augusta, Me., 1904), p. 235.

12. *Minutes of the Common Council of the City of New York, 1675-1766* (New York, 1905), pp. 121-123; *Laws, Statutes, Ordinances and Constitutions of the City of New York* (New York, 1731), pp. 27-29. Quoted in Janet B. Donegan, "Midwifery in America, 1760-1860: A Study in Medicine and Morality" (unpublished Ph.D. dissertation, Syracuse University, 1972), pp. 9-10.

13. Kate Campbell Hurd-Mead, *A History of Women in Medicine* (Haddam, Conn., 1938), p. 391.

14. Version is the changing of the fetus in utero. In a normal labor the head presents itself first. When another part of the anatomy, such as an arm or buttock is present, version must be performed in order to manipulate the fetus into a cephalic (head first) or podalic (feet first) position.

15. Embryulcia is the extraction of the fetus from the uterus. Colonial physicians performed embryulcia if the fetus died in utero. If the mother's life was in danger, embryulcia was sometimes performed while the fetus was still alive. Embryulcia usually involved decapitation, amputation, or perforation of the skull.

16. Richard Wertz and Dorothy Wertz, "Lying-in, A History of Childbirth in America: Its Technologies and Social Relations" (Boston, unpublished manuscript [1974]), [2].

17. Susanna Müller, 1756-1815. "An Old German Midwife's Record." Edited by M. D. Learned and C. F. Bride, [n.p., n.d.]. Located at the Library of the College of Physicians of Philadelphia; Nash, *History of Augusta,* p. 235.

18. Wertz, "Lying-in," Chapter 1. Catherine M. Scholten, " 'On the Importance of the Obstetrick Art': Changing Customs of Childbirth in America, 1760-1825," forthcoming article in *William and Mary Quarterly.*

19. Herbert Thoms, *Our Obstetric Heritage: The Story of Safe Childbirth* (Hamden, Conn., 1960), pp. 7-9, 16.

20. Although it is possible that there were male midwives who were not also physicians, no evidence has been uncovered to this effect. During the colonial era, however, it was relatively easy for a man to acquire a physician's reputation. Donegan, "Midwifery in America," pp. 17-18, 35-39, passim.

21. Goodell, "When and Why," 382.

22. Howard D. King, "The Evolution of the Male Midwife, with Some Remarks on the Obstetrical Literature of Other Ages," *American Journal of Obstetrics and the Diseases of Women and Children,* 77 (February 1918), 185. William F. Mengert, "The Origin of the Male Midwife," *Annals of Medical History,* 4 (September 1932), 453.

23. Graham, *Eternal Eve,* pp. 111, 112; Donegan, "Midwifery in America," pp. 21-23.

24. Graham, *Eternal Eve,* pp. 151-153; Donegan, "Midwifery in America, pp. 26-28.

25. Quoted in King, "Evolution," pp. 185-186.

26. Donegan, "Midwifery in America," p. 28.

27. *Pennsylvania Gazette,* January 31, 1765. Quoted in Betsy E. Corner, *William Shippen, Jr., Pioneer in American Medical Education* (Philadelphia, 1951), p. 103.

28. Richard H. Shryock, *Medicine in America: Historical Essays* (Baltimore, 1966), p. 181.

29. The most thorough account of the eighteenth-century conflict between midwives and male midwives can be found in Donegan, "Midwifery in America," pp. 1-67.

30. Henry B. Shafer, *The American Medical Profession 1783-1850* (New York, 1936), pp. 13-19. The four schools were the University of Pennsylvania Medical School (College of Philadelphia, 1765), Columbia University Medical School (King's College, 1768), Harvard Medical School (Massachusetts Medical College, 1783), and Dartmouth Medical School (1798).

31. Valentine Seaman, *The Midwives' Monitor and Mother's Mirror* (New York, 1800), pp. 101-102. Quoted in Donegan, "Midwifery in America," p. 63.

32. For additional information on Seaman and Bard, see Donegan, "Midwifery in America," pp. 60-68; Thoms, *Our Obstetric Heritage*, pp. 71-74. Bard also maintained that physicians employed the forceps too freely.

33. Donegan, "Midwifery in America," pp. 51-54.

34. *The Essex Gazette* (Salem), July 14, 1772. Quoted in Donegan, "Midwifery in America," p. 54.

35. Richard H. Shryock, *Medical Licensing in America, 1650-1965* (Baltimore, 1967), p. 103. Thoms, *Our Obstetric Heritage*, p. 140.

36. Thomas Ewell, *Letters to Ladies, Detailing Important Information Concerning Themselves and Infants* (Philadelphia, 1817), pp. 26, 27. Quoted in Donegan, "Midwifery in America," p. 131.

37. *An Appeal to the Medical Society of Rhode-Island, in Behalf of Woman to be Restored to her Natural Rights as "Midwife" and Elevated by Education to be the Physician of her Own Sex* (1851), p. 4.

38. Donegan, "Midwifery in America," pp. 115-116. At least one early feminist did bemoan the declining status of the midwife. Mary Wollstonecraft argued in *A Vindication of the Rights of Woman* (New York, 1967; reprint of 1792 edition) that women should be encouraged

to study the art of healing and be physicians as well as nurses. And, midwifery, decency seems to allot to them [women] though I am afraid the word midwife in our dictionaries will soon give place to *accoucheur*, and one proof of the former delicacy of the sex be effaced from the language. (221-222)

39. *An Appeal to the Medical Society of Rhode-Island*, p. 5.

40. John Van Pelt Quackenbush, *An Address Delivered before the Students of the Albany Medical College, Introductory to the Course on Obstetrics, November 5, 1855* (Albany, 1855), p. 4. Quoted in Donegan, "Midwifery in America," p. 240.

41. The standard history of the New England Female Medical College is Frederick C. Waite, *History of the New England Female Medical College,*

1848-1874 (Boston, 1950). For a more critical view of Gregory, see Mary Roth Walsh, *"Doctors Wanted: No Women Need Apply." Sexual Barriers in the Medical Profession, 1835-1975* (New Haven, Conn., 1977), pp. 35-75.

42. *Boston Medical and Surgical Journal,* 37 (September 1847), 184-185. Quoted in Donegan, "Midwifery in America," pp. 154-155.

43. Walter Channing, *Remarks on the Employment of Females as Practitioners in Midwifery* (Boston, 1820), pp. 4-7; Donegan, "Midwifery in America," pp. 242-244. Two especially useful articles on nineteenth-century attitudes toward women are Barbara Welter,"The Cult of True Womanhood 1820-1860," *American Quarterly,* 18 (Summer 1966), 151-174; and Carroll Smith-Rosenberg and Charles Rosenberg, "The Female Animal: Medical and Biological Views of Woman and Her Role in Nineteenth-Century America," *Journal of American History,* 60 (September 1973), 332-356.

44. Packard, *History of Medicine,* II, 1125-1127.

45. The monthly nurse was a woman who was hired to perform medical and housewifely duties. Her employment began at the onset of labor and lasted for about one month. She did not, however, deliver the baby unless the physician was late in arriving at the home of the parturient woman.

See, for example, Pye Henry Chavasse, *Woman as a Wife and Mother* (Philadelphia, 1870), pp. 189-193; John H. Dye, *Painless Childbirth; or Healthy Mothers and Healthy Children* (Silver Creek, N.Y., 1884), pp. 156-157; Anna M. Fullerton, *A Handbook of Obstetrical Nursing for Nurses, Students and Mothers* (Philadelphia, 1890), pp. 65-82; George H. Napheys, *The Physical Life of Woman: Advice to the Maiden, Wife and Mother* (Philadelphia, 1890), pp. 244-245; Prudence B. Saur, *Maternity: A Book for Every Wife and Mother* (Chicago, 1891), pp. 217-219; Alice B. Stockham, *Tokology: A Book for Every Woman* (Chicago, 1885), p. 163; Tullio Suzzara Verdi, *Maternity: A Popular Treatise for Young Wives and Mothers* (Philadelphia, 1885), p. 131.

2

The Beginnings of Obstetric Specialization

A handful of nineteenth-century physicians were responsible for a variety of medical discoveries that served to raise the status of obstetrics and gynecology and discredit the work of midwives. Interestingly, it was the work of a few rural physicians that propelled the United States into a leadership position in the field of gynecology. For example, in 1809, a Kentucky physician, Emphraim McDowell, performed the first successful ovariotomy. More important were the discoveries of J. Marion Sims, often referred to as the "father of modern gynecology." Sims received his medical education at the Medical College of South Carolina and Jefferson Medical College in Philadelphia. He then moved to Alabama where he began practicing medicine. By experimenting on slave women, Sims was able to develop a cure for the vesico-vaginal fistula in 1849.[1] He also designed the curved vaginal speculum, and he established the Woman's Hospital of New York City in 1855, the first hospital in the United States devoted exclusively to the diseases of women and children.[2] Another country physician, Robert Battey of Rome, Georgia, invented the "normal ovariotomy" in 1872. Battey called it a "normal ovariotomy" because he recommended the removal of the ovaries for non-ovarian causes, such as "neurosis, insanity, abnormal menstruation, and practically anything untoward in female behavior." Clitoridectomy, although not invented by an American, was practiced in this country from 1867 until 1904 or perhaps as late as 1925.[3]

An assortment of obstetric achievements appeared concurrently with the gynecologic discoveries of the nineteenth century. The use of anesthesia in surgery in the late 1840s substantially altered the birth process for many women. Dr. Walter Channing, who in 1848 published a *Treatise on Etherization in Childbirth*, was instrumental in convincing physicians to use ether in both difficult and normal labors. In 1853, the entire world took note of the fact that Queen Victoria was administered chloroform during childbirth. The question of the safety of anesthesia in childbirth caused some physicians to continue to disapprove of its use. In addition, many of the early anesthetic critics were opposed to alleviating the pain of childbirth because they maintained that suffering was what caused a woman to develop love for her offspring. Pain in childbirth was also believed to be ordained by God as evidenced in Genesis 3:16: ". . . in pain you shall bring forth children. . . ."[4]

Another event of the 1840s that eventually revolutionized the process of childbirth was the discovery of the contagious nature of puerperal (childbed) fever. Two physicians, Oliver Wendell Holmes and Ignaz Semmelweis, an Austrian, independently of each other developed the theory that the puerperal germ traveled from patient to patient by way of the hands of the attending physician. Both men were ridiculed by their contemporaries for suggesting that a physician's hands might be dirty, and many doctors adamantly refused to wash their hands before examining parturient women. Holmes and Semmelweis were eventually vindicated when physicians began to realize that the late nineteenth-century bacteriological discoveries of Louis Pasteur and Joseph Lister were applicable to the practice of obstetrics.[5] The use of antiseptic techniques also made obstetric and gynecologic operations, such as the cesarean section and hysterectomy, much safer.[6]

The gap between trained physicians and midwives continued to grow as other gynecologic and obstetric discoveries were made. The use of ergot to induce uterine contractions was introduced into the United States by Dr. John Stearns of New York in 1808. In the 1820s, the stethoscope was applied to the woman's abdomen in order that the fetal heartbeat might be heard. Instruments were developed that could dilate the cervix so that other instruments, such as the uterine sound, could be introduced into the uterus. Studies dealing with ectopic (extra-uterine) gestation were undertaken. In the 1870s, it was discovered that ophthalmia neonatorum could be prevented by applying silver nitrate to the eyes of the newborn infant.[7] By the early twentieth century, X-rays were providing precise pelvic measurements.

The gradual acceptance of clinical instruction in obstetrics gave physicians another advantage over midwives that they had not, heretofore, enjoyed. In 1850, Dr. James Platt White, professor of obstetrics at Buffalo Medical College, evoked a furor among his colleagues and the general public when he introduced the practice of "demonstrative midwifery" in his classroom. For the first time in American history, medical students were able to view the birth of a baby. Physicians who supported the midwife immediately attacked this practice as unnecessary and offensive. Defenders of demonstrative midwifery pointed out that clinical instruction in obstetrics had been practiced in Europe at least since the days of Smellie.[8]

The growth of dispensaries and the rise of hospitals reinforced the view that demonstrative midwifery was advisable. Moreover, the establishment of the Woman's Hospital of New York City by J. Marion Sims in 1855 was the first of several specialized hospitals for women founded in the United States during the second half of the nineteenth century.[9] Despite these developments, clinical instruction in obstetrics won acceptance slowly. Dr. J. Whitridge Williams, the leading figure in American obstetrics during the first three decades of the twentieth century, observed only two deliveries before graduating from the University of Maryland in 1888. Williams's lack of clinical observation, however, did not prevent him from winning his alma mater's obstetric prize.[10]

During the second half of the nineteenth century, the American medical profession began to take concrete steps to insure that obstetrics would eventually receive its due recognition. In 1859, for example, the American Medical Association designated practical medicine and obstetrics as one of the four scientific sections of the association.[11] The *American Journal of Obstetrics*, the first specialized medical journal published in the Untied States, was founded in 1868. The establishment of the American Gynecological Society

in 1876 and the American Association of Obstetricians and Gynecologists in 1888 also advanced the tenet that obstetrics was a complicated specialty which only the physician was capable of pursuing.[12]

By the late nineteenth century, the middle and upper classes were
beginning to embrace the view that childbirth was a disease that
could most properly be controlled by the use of instruments, drugs,
and surgery.[13] Physicians, who during the early years of the nineteenth century had defended the midwife against the male midwife
in the name of decency and morality, now rarely spoke out in her
behalf. Indeed, the male-midwifery debate was laid to rest once the
medical profession and the public began to accept the idea that
childbirth was a complicated medical specialty requiring the services
of the highly trained physician. The well-being and safety of the
parturient woman were deemed more important than the preserva-
tion of decency and morality in the lying-in chamber.[14]

Significantly, the medical profession appeared to show only
peripheral interest in the present and future status of the midwife
during the latter decades of the nineteenth century. Occasionally,
medical journals published articles on the midwife. The question
now being debated, however, was whether or not midwives were
capable of serving as competent birth attendants. The growth of
medical professionalism and new discoveries in the field of obstetrics
had ushered in the rudimentary stage of what would eventually
become a heated and vociferous debate over the midwife's status in
American society. Not until 1910 would the debate reach full force.
Nevertheless, the arguments developed during the last two decades
of the nineteenth century are important because they provide a
preview of what is to come.

For example, in 1884, Dr. T. H. Manley delivered a paper to the
New York State Medical Association in which he summed up many
of the arguments that were voiced by midwife proponents during
the second and third decades of the twentieth century. Manley
believed that trained and properly educated midwives were capable
of attending "normal confinements." He congratulated them for
not using ergot or forceps to speed up the process of labor. At the
same time, he was quite distressed over the fact that there were so
few training programs for midwives in the United States, and he
was hopeful that New York City would lead the way in midwife

education and training. While Manley insisted that "social and physiological reasons" prevented women from becoming successful physicians, he was certain that they were "well calculated to act as midwives." Finally, he attempted to allay the fears of those doctors who were concerned that midwives might reduce their revenue. He labeled this fear as "more imaginary than real" because the classes which depend on midwives are not "able to fairly remunerate a physician for his services."[15]

C. S. Bacon, professor of obstetrics at Chicago Polyclinic, was another late nineteenth-century defender of the midwife whose arguments were often reiterated during the 1910-1930 era. In a paper which he presented to the Section on Obstetrics and Diseases of Women at the 1897 annual meeting of the American Medical Association, Bacon also expressed concern over the lack of training programs for midwives. He felt that their education and regulation could be most effectively handled by the various state boards of health. He opposed replacing them with lying-in charities because the patients who employ midwives "are not paupers who demand gratuitous services and they will not allow themselves to be used as clinical material." Bacon did not view the midwife and the physician as antagonists. He argued that on the contrary "the midwife will come to regard the physician not as her enemy but as her counselor and helper in difficulties, and the physician will learn to appreciate and respect the properly qualified midwife."[16]

The most prevalent argument expressed by late nineteenth-century midwife critics was that childbirth was a potentially dangerous phenomenon that often required the services of the well-qualified medical practitioner. In language characteristic of other anti-midwife physicians, Dr. W. S. Smith insisted, in a paper which he read at the 1895 annual session of the Medical and Chirurgical Faculty of Maryland, that parturition was not a natural process, because "no matter how naturally or with what comparative ease a woman may pass through the confinement, she is in all cases a wounded woman, presenting to us, not only the extremely sensitive and receptive uterine wound, but numerous tears, contusions, and abrasions of the genital tract, . . ." Although Smith was highly critical of the "gross manipulations and hazardous practices of ignorant and officious midwives," he reluctantly conceded that steps to train them, along the lines established in Germany and England, might be possible.[17] Smith's remarks apparently did not reach a very large audience, for ten years later, W. C. Gewin, a physician from Birmingham, Alabama, was credited with writing the same paper identical in content as well as title.[18]

H. J. Garrigues, a New York City obstetrician, was also critical of the work performed by midwives. In an article published in *Medical News* in 1898, he argued that midwives were "inveterate quacks" who treat "disturbances during the puerpery, later gynecologic diseases, then diseases of children, and are finally consulted in regard to almost anything. They never acknowledge their ignorance, and are always willing to give some advice." Garrigues was basically opposed to training programs and schools for midwives. He urged the United States to "form the vanguard in a war of extermination against the pestiferous remnant of the pre-antiseptic days, midwives, and schools of midwifery." He admitted that the present midwife situation with regard to education and legal recognition was chaotic, but he preferred this chaos "for the simple reason that it cannot last forever, and that it must lead to the enactment of a law by which midwifery, as all other branches of medical practice, is exclusively placed in the hands of the medical profession, where it belongs."[19]

Garrigues also went to great lengths to "prove" that there was "a superabundance of medical men" in the United States who were in great need of additional obstetric cases. He calculated that in 1890 there was one physician for every 150 women of childbearing age. Since women, by liberal estimates, gave birth to only four children during the thirty-year childbearing period, Garrigues figured that there were "about nineteen confinements every year for each physician in the United States." He concluded that midwives were unnecessary because physicians, alone, could easily take care of all the obstetric cases. He quickly added that analogies could not be drawn with European countries where there were far fewer doctors ranging from 1 in 2,000 to 1 in 6,000 of the population.[20]

By and large, however, late nineteenth-century physicians appeared to be indifferent to the midwife. They assumed that the parturient woman would hire both a physician and monthly nurse for her confinement.[21] Thus, they made few attempts to establish training programs or regulatory legislation for midwives.[22] The growth of medical professionalism and new discoveries in the field of obstetrics seemed to insure that American midwives would eventually be displaced by physicians. Consequently, most late nineteenth-century medical practitioners complacently ignored the midwife.

NOTES

1. Prolonged labor sometimes results in a condition known as the vesico-vaginal fistula. This condition occurs when the head of the fetus presses against the roof of the vagina in such a way and to such extent, that the tissues become gangrenous, die off, and produce an opening, most often between the bladder and the vagina. A vesico-vaginal fistula involves a constant leakage of urine, producing irritation, excoriation, and in numerous cases, infections of the urogenital area involving the thighs and the perenium. Furthermore, such an infected patient carries with her a constant odor which renders her repulsive to others and produces unfortunate psychological reactions. Until 1849, when Sims developed his cure, all attempts at treating the vesico-vaginal fistula had been unsuccessful.

2. For more information on Sims, see Seale Harris, *Woman's Surgeon: The Life Story of J. Marion Sims* (New York, 1950); G. J. Barker-Benfield, *The Horrors of the Half-Known Life: Male Attitudes Toward Woman and Sexuality in Nineteenth-Century America* (New York, 1976), pp. 80-132. The Harris biography is filled with praise for Sims, while Barker-Benfield argues that Sims's desire to repair the vesico-vaginal fistula and cure other gynecologic disorders grew out of "his fundamental desire to shape women, control them, and thereby to foster his own immortality." (109)

3. Ben Barker-Benfield, "The Spermatic Economy: A Nineteenth Century View of Sexuality," *Feminist Studies*, 1 (1970), 59-60.

4. Herbert Thoms, *Chapters in American Obstetrics* (Springfield, Ill., 1933), p. 10.

5. Walter Radcliffe, *Milestones in Midwifery* (Bristol, England, 1967), pp. 88-89.

6. The first cesarean section was recorded by the ancient Hebrews in the *Talmud*. As late as the mid-nineteenth century, the death rate from this operation ranged from 50 to 85 percent. The hazards associated with the operation meant that few physicians were willing to attempt it unless the parturient woman was almost moribund. The development of a technique to close the uterine incision with sutures in 1882 and the application of antiseptic procedures prompted physicians to perform cesarean sections

on women who were not moribund. Consequently, the mortality rate associated with cesarean sections significantly declined during the late nineteenth and early twentieth centuries. Theodore Cianfrani, *A Short History of Obstetrics and Gynecology* (Springfield, Ill., 1960), pp. 363, 365. Irving S. Cutter and Henry R. Viets, *A Short History of Midwifery* (Philadelphia, 1964), pp. 154-155.

7. Ophthalmia neonatorum is an eye infection sometimes found in newborn infants which is usually caused by a gonorrheal discharge from the mother's genitals. Until the discovery that silver nitrate served as a prophylaxis against opthalmia neonatorum, many infants were totally blinded by this disease.

8. Janet B. Donegan, "Midwifery in America, 1760-1860: A Study in Medicine and Morality" (unpublished Ph.D. dissertation, Syracuse University, 1972), pp. 26, 211.

9. Some of the most notable early hospitals established exclusively for women and children include the following: New York Infirmary for Women and Children (1857); New England Hospital for Women and Children (1862); Chicago Hospital for Women and Children (1870); Sloane Maternity Hospital of the College of Physicians and Surgeons of New York City (1888).

10. Harold Speert, *The Sloane Hospital Chronicle* (Philadelphia, 1963), p. 80.

11. The other three scientific sections of the American Medical Association were (1) anatomy and physiology, (2) chemistry and materia medica, and (3) surgery. Susan Crawford, *Digest of Official Actions: American Medical Association, 1846-1958* ([Chicago], 1959), p. 643.

12. Richard B. Morris, ed., *Encyclopedia of American History* (New York, 1965), p. 574; Rosemary Stevens, *American Medicine and the Public Interest* (New Haven, Conn., 1971), p. 46.

13. Dorothy Wertz and Richard Wertz, "Childbirth as Disease" (unpublished paper read at the Second Berkshire Conference on the History of Women, Radcliffe College, Cambridge, Mass., October 26, 1974), p. 13.

14. Some parturient women were, of course, attended by female physicians. In fact, approximately 200 to 300 women held the M.D. degree by 1860. Most male physicians, however, supported a variety of measures aimed at preventing women from becoming successful medical practitioners. Donegan, "Midwifery in America," pp. 202-263. See also Mary Roth Walsh, *"Doctors Wanted: No Women Need Apply." Sexual Barriers in the Medical Profession, 1835-1975* (New Haven, Conn., 1977), pp. 106-146.

15. T. H. Manley, "Women as Midwives," *Transactions of the New York State Medical Association,* 1 (1884), 371, 372, 373-374, 375. See also C. A.

Von Ramdohr, "Midwifery and Midwife," *Medical Record*, 3 (December 1897), 882-883.

16. C. S. Bacon, "The Midwife Question in America," *Journal of the American Medical Association*, 29 (November 1897), 1092.

17. W. S. Smith, "Careless and Unscientific Midwifery, with Special Reference to Some Features of the Work of Midwives," *Maryland Medical Journal*, 33 (1895-1896), 148. For similar views, see Robert C. Eve, "Licensing of Midwives," *Charlotte (North Carolina) Medical Journal*, 6 (1895), 990-995; L. C. Wadsworth, "The Midwife and Midwifery," *American Practitioner and News*, 26 (1898), 209-212.

18. W. C. Gewin, "Careless and Unscientific Midwifery with Special References to Some Features of the Work of Midwives," *Alabama Medical Journal*, 18 (1905-1906), 629-635.

19. H. J. Garrigues, "Midwives," *Medical News*, 72 (1898), 233, 235.

20. Ibid., 235. See also J. H. Pryor, "The Status of the Midwife in Buffalo," *New York Medical Journal*, 11 (August 1884), 131.

21. See Chapter 1, note 45.

22. White House Conference on Child Health and Protection, *Obstetric Education* (New York, 1932), pp. 178-192; Louis S. Reed, *Midwives, Chiropodists, and Optometrists: Their Place in Medical Care* (Chicago, 1932), pp. 15-16; Richard H. Shryock, *Medical Licensing in America, 1650-1965* (Baltimore, 1967), pp. 49-50.

3

Forgotten Women: American Midwives at the Turn of the Twentieth Century

At the turn of the century, midwives and physicians attended about an equal number of births. Indeed, although statistics relating to the number of early twentieth-century midwives are not always reliable, conservative estimates indicate that as late as 1910 at least 50 percent of all births were attended by midwives.[1] Southern black families relied heavily on midwives. In 1918, 87.9 percent of all Negro births in Mississippi were attended by midwives. Immigrant women, especially those newly arrived from southern and eastern Europe, also used midwives. A 1908 study revealed that 86 percent of all Italian-American births in Chicago were reported by midwives. In isolated, rural areas of the United States, a friend or relative often acted as a midwife in the absence of the doctor. Moreover, there was no clear demarcation line between the woman who acted in the official capacity of a midwife once or twice a year and the neighbor who occasionally came to the aid of a friend in need.[2]

Although the early twentieth-century midwife was numerically significant, middle- and upper-class white Americans had little firsthand contact with her. The woman of wealthy or moderate means usually enlisted both a physician and monthly nurse for the confinement period. A growing number of well-to-do women were even choosing to have their babies in hospitals in order that they might be able to employ obstetric specialists. Hospitalization for childbirth, however, was the exception, and in 1900 the vast majority of all births occurred in the home.[3]

Only the very poor, who accepted public or private charities, and the well-to-do, who could afford competent obstetricians, went to the hospital. Families with moderate incomes could not pay the high price of hospital deliveries. This predicament caused several prominent physicians to argue that the very poor received better obstetric care than "the most self-respecting element in the community; the wives of clerks, small store-keepers, artisans, book-keepers, and similar employees whose weekly wages range from $15.00 to $30.00." Prohibitive fees were not the only factor limiting the number of hospital births. Just as important was the widespread belief that the hospital was a disease-ridden institution where people went to die. Surgical operations and other types of obstetric interference were also closely associated with hospital delivery. Thus, poor women often preferred to pay the small fee of the midwife rather than enter a charity hospital where they allegedly would be subjected to experimentation and obstetric interference.[4]

Clearly, many immigrant and black women were attracted to midwives because of the small fees they charged. The average fee of the midwife from Waterbury, Connecticut, in 1913 was $8, while the physician charged between $15 and $25. In rural Mississippi in 1916 the midwife's fee ranged between $5 and $10, depending on the difficulty of the case, the distance from the patient, and the ability of the family to pay. Often, informal arrangements were made for payment in chickens, pigs, grain, or on a neighborly give-and-take-basis. One black Mississippi midwife even admitted that she charged more for boys than girls because "boys are harder to handle and mothers want them more." In contrast, Mississippi physicians charged between $10 and $15 for normal deliveries, plus additional fees for prenatal and postnatal visits.[5]

Midwives not only charged substantially less than did physicians, but they also provided a variety of services that general practitioners did not offer. The midwife served as the birth attendant, nurse, and housekeeper. In addition to caring for the mother and newborn infant, she also cleaned the house, prepared the meals, and looked after other children in the family for from three to ten days after the birth of the baby. Women who used midwives were well aware that they were receiving services not offered by physicians. A 1924 Texas midwifery survey revealed that many women preferred midwives because they were "really worth more." One woman pointed out that the midwife "did my washing and charged only $5." Another stated that she paid $7.50 for three and one-half days of service. Thus, the midwife combined the duties of the physician and monthly nurse for less than one-half the fee usually charged by the physician.[6] It is likely that midwives were expected to perform housewifely functions because society had traditionally perceived women as wives and mothers.

The preference of immigrants for midwives was reinforced by the fact that it was a long-established European tradition to have them serve as attendants at birth. Hence, most midwives in Europe held high positions in the community and were usually well trained and well supervised. When immigrant women arrived in America, they continued to employ midwives even though very few provisions for their training and regulation existed in the United States at the turn of the twentieth century.[7]

The fact that the midwife spoke the language of the parturient woman was also important. Physicians, in contrast, were often unable to communicate in any language other than English. Most importantly, immigrant families employed midwives because there was a "strong sense of shame [associated] with permitting a man to attend a woman in confinement." The degree to which various immigrant groups opposed men in the lying-in chamber varied. Italians and Lithuanians were singled out as being especially hostile to male accoucheurs. Almost all contemporary observers agreed that the immigrants' dislike for men in the lying-in chamber had a great deal to do with the popularity of midwives.[8]

Because middle- and upper-class Americans no longer shared this view, they were generally unsympathetic to the stance of the immigrants. They argued that the midwife was not a native product of America and not suitable to the American situation. She was characterized as "a remnant of barbaric times, a blot on our civilization, which ought to be wiped out as soon as possible."[9] Ironically, the American male-midwifery controversy had reached its peak only sixty years earlier. At the turn of the century, many middle-

and upper-class white Americans appeared to have forgotten that they, too, had once defiantly opposed the presence of men in the lying-in chamber.

Black women also expressed a dislike for male birth attendants. The 1924 survey of midwifery in Texas disclosed that many black women were "ashamed to have a man at that time" and that they preferred the midwife because she "is a woman and will be more help than [the] doctor." One woman stated, "I am used to women and not strange men like doctors." The Texas women also indicated that it was traditional to use midwives. Another woman remarked that she "never knew anything else but a midwife." A frequent explanation given for employing midwives was that "everybody else had them around here." Another woman commented that the midwife was "just handed down from slavery times." Black women also preferred midwives because of their easy accessibility. Southern physicians usually lived in the towns and cities and often had to travel long distances in order to reach the parturient women. In contrast, midwives were scattered throughout the rural South. Accordingly, Texas women chose midwives because "way out in the country doctors charge too much."[10]

Any attempt to present a composite picture of early twentieth-century midwives is complicated by the fact that no diaries, letters, autobiographies, or other manuscript materials of turn-of-the-century midwives have been uncovered.[11] Moreover, midwifery legislation was almost nonexistent prior to 1910, and the few regulations that were enacted were usually not enforced. Thus, little information with regard to the practices of midwives can be garnered from legal sources.[12] In addition, much of the existing information about them was written by hostile observers: both northern and southern writers frequently portrayed midwives as "dirty," "ignorant," and "evil."[13]

Northern observers were especially concerned about the growing number of midwives who were believed to be performing illegal abortions. One early twentieth-century study of midwives in New York City reported that 176 of 500 midwives under investigation had participated in such "criminal work." A similar study of Chicago midwives classified one-third of them as "criminal." The Chicago study also disclosed that physicians often supported the "criminal midwives" by falsifying death certificates for them.[14]

Southern reports dwelled on the superstitions and folklore of the "granny" midwives, which were "so gross in many cases as to rival voodooism." One contemporary observer related the story of the "granny" who always asked for whiskey for the baby's scalp. When the liquor was procured, several ounces went to "her melancholy soul" while only a few drops found their way to the baby's scalp. Black midwives in Maryland were reported to treat hemorrhaging by placing either ice or hot potatoes in the hand of the parturient woman. Many "grannies" believed that a difficult labor might be made easier by throwing hot coals on hen feathers and placing the ashes under the prospective mother's bed. A popular remedy for hastening labor was to give tea made from the dirt dauber's nest to the pregnant woman. The southern black midwife was also characterized as an old woman who was qualified for nothing except "catching babies." A favorite quotation included in studies about southern midwives came from an eighty-year-old "granny" who supposedly stated, "I am too old to clean; too weak to wash; too blind to sew; but, thank God! I can still put my neighbors to bed."[15]

Even studies conducted by the United States Children's Bureau, which was generally sympathetic to midwives, reported considerable ignorance and superstition among "grannies." An investigation of maternity care in rural Mississippi for the years 1916-1918 reported that two-thirds of the black midwives were illiterate. Although the white midwives were "superior" to their black counterparts, they "did not differ either in training or practice from the Negro midwives." Nine-tenths of the rural Mississippi midwives, most of whom were black, used no antiseptics. Only the "more intelligent ones" realized that puerperal fever was caused by uncleanliness, and many midwives continued to adhere to the old custom of not changing the bed coverings for at least three days after the birth. The report also revealed that only three of the eighty-seven Mississippi midwives interviewed put drops of silver nitrate in the newborn infant's eyes, although this was required by state law. A similar study of maternity care in the north Georgia mountains for the years 1916-1918 also disclosed that midwives were "steeped in the superstitions and practices of a bygone generation." Significantly, most of the Georgia mountain midwives were white. Although the majority of the accounts of southern midwives focused on the "ignorance" and "superstition" of the black "grannies," contemporary reports also indicated that white midwives were sorely lacking in the basic knowledge required of competent attendants at birth.[16]

Very few satisfactory training programs for midwives existed at the turn of the twentieth century. This helps to explain why contemporary observers frequently characterized them as "dirty," "ignorant," and "evil." In most instances, those midwives who wanted to learn more about pregnancy and parturition could not obtain competent, inexpensive training. Between 1916 and 1918, for example, Mississippi midwives expressed an interest in having public health nurses advise them, but there were no nurses available for that purpose. Some southern midwives served apprenticeships with physicians. Usually, "grannies" were taught by their mothers or older midwives. Like the colonial midwife, most of the knowledge of the southern "granny" was a result of firsthand experience and observation.[17]

Many black women also felt that it was necessary to be "called by the Lord." In a recent interview, Elizabeth Singleton, a 104-year-old black midwife from Wayne County, Georgia, underscored the importance of the "calling." In recounting her experiences as a midwife, Singleton remarked

The good Lord taught me how to catch babies. . . . I don't know how many babies I caught; must have been more than 1,000, both black and white babies. . . . When I was catching babies, I would pray for you. I would ask the Lord to help you and to help me to take care of you. I've prayed so hard, and my soul would be so full of joy. . . . I never used any instruments. I worked with doctors. I used herbs. I always gave new mothers ginger tea to keep their blood from clotting. I stopped catching babies when the law said I had to stop—I guess it was sometime in the '40's.[18]

A few schools for midwives did exist in the northeastern and midwestern areas of the United States at the turn of the twentieth century, but the course of instruction provided at most of them was totally inadequate. Early twentieth-century midwife studies concurred in the opinion that the schools were "veritable diploma mills run for revenue only, usually by some conscienceless physician who receives lucrative returns for a minimum outlay of time and trouble." The fees charged by the physicians were, in fact, exorbitant. The average cost of a six-month course of study in Chicago in 1907 was $100-$175. This fee usually included nothing more than lectures for three to four hours each week in the physician's back office. Often the instructor required no textbooks and provided no clinical instruction for his students. Schools for midwives in New York City provided the same type of low-quality education. A 1907 study of New York City midwives disclosed that some women who could neither read nor write held midwifery diplomas from New York schools. They had "earned" their diplomas because they could afford the tuition charge of $66. Four such diploma mills were known to exist in New York City in 1907. Graduates of these schools recounted the dread and fear they suffered as they went to their first cases without the supervision of either a physician or experienced midwife. The quality of the education in the New York City schools was so deplorable that the author of the 1907 study concluded that the "eighty-eight midwives who had no diplomas [were] quite as efficient and capable as the 209 who held those worthless New York diplomas."[19]

In both Chicago and New York City, there was also evidence of collusion between the physician-instructor and the midwife. Arrangements were reportedly made in which the poorly trained midwife agreed to call on her former instructor for assistance during difficult labors. Thus, she was protected, and the physician received an additional source of income. On other occasions, the midwife might enlist the aid of the physician on the pretext that something had gone wrong. The physician would respond by using forceps or performing other services that the midwife could not render. He would then share the high fee he charged for the "complicated" labor with the cooperating midwife.[20]

It would, however, be a mistake to leave the impression that all turn-of-the-century midwives were poorly trained. Newly arrived immigrant midwives were often graduates of excellent European midwifery schools. Of course, most Americans were not familiar enough with the European situation to know whether or not the foreign diplomas displayed by the midwives were from reputable schools. Moreover, the European-trained midwife often became careless in her practice once she arrived in the United States where few rules and regulations existed. It was also economically impossible for her to compete with the American idea of the midwife and still maintain the high standards she had been taught in Europe.[21]

Interestingly enough, Mormon midwives were also well trained. During the latter half of the nineteenth century, Mormon husbands encouraged their wives to study midwifery in order to save expenses. For example, Zina D. H. Young, the wife of Brigham Young, delivered hundreds of babies including her husband's more than fifty-five children by other women. The widespread opposition to the practice of polygamy made it essential for Mormon women to be trained as midwives. Throughout the 1880s and 1890s, Mormon midwives observed professional secrecy in an attempt to prevent United States deputies from tracing the sources of polygamous activity. They received most of their training while serving apprenticeships under Mormon physicians. Some midwives also attended medical colleges, such as the Woman's Medical College of Pennsylvania. When formal training programs were not available, Mormon midwives took up self-study and went "as thoroughly as possible into the subject from every angle that . . . [they] would be required to meet. . . ."[22]

There were even a few American schools that provided adequate training programs for midwives. In 1883, the New York State Supreme Court granted the College of Midwifery of New York City the right to confer the diploma of Graduate in Midwifery. The college advertised that it was "the only regular institution in America incorporated for the purpose of conferring on women the diploma of Graduate in Midwifery." The faculty consisted of seven physicians. The lone woman, Sarah E. Post, served as professor of physiology. She was also the attending physician to the Out-door Department of the New York Infirmary for Women and Children. The respectability of the college was further enhanced by the fact that Dr. J. Marion Sims agreed to serve as consulting gynecologist to the Woman's Infirmary and Maternity Home of the College of Midwifery. Sims's death in 1883 prevented him from serving in this capacity.[23]

The course of instruction at the college included lectures, recitations, and demonstrations in English, German, French, and Spanish for a three-month period. This was followed by three months of practical work at the Metropolitan Dispensary for Women and the

Woman's Infirmary and Maternity Home. The cost of the six-month course was $105. If a candidate failed to pass the final examination, she could enroll in the college a second time by paying a fee of $30. Fourteen students attended the first session, and ten satisfactorily completed the course. The faculty believed that the "interests of the institution and the community would be better served by teaching a limited number thoroughly and well, rather than send out a large class unqualified."[24]

In the original bulletin announcing the opening of the college, the members of the Board of Trustees explained why such a school was necessary. Predictably, they pointed to the lack of training programs for midwives in the United States. They included extensive quotations from the congratulatory and commendatory notices that had appeared in some of the leading medical journals of America. These notices reiterated that the United States had "thus far . . . been desitute of any adequate provision . . ." for the education of midwives. The trustees also defended the concept of formal training for midwives on the grounds "that it teaches, what, by experience, had been found to cover the sphere of woman's usefulness in medicine." They argued that women were especially suited for training in midwifery, but that they were not, in most instances, capable of undergoing the "whole curriculum of surgery, pharmacy, materia medica, jurisprudence, etc." The failure of female medical schools to attract large numbers of students was used as proof that women did not have the ability to become regular practitioners of medicine. Moreover, the trustees also believed that it was "not necessary to lay open the entire subject of obstetrics to the midwife. On the contrary, her practice should be strictly limited; the knowledge imparted serving mainly to indicate to her when the accoucheur is to be called in, and that the office of midwife is to attend women in natural labor."[25]

The Playfair School of Midwifery in Chicago, Illinois, was another institution that provided quality education for midwives. It was established in 1896 for the purpose of interesting

such a class of women in this work that by proper opportunities we will remove the present prevailing prejudice against the midwife and finally restore her to her proper reputable position in the profession, not as a competitor to the physician, but able to conduct normal labor with safety, and, . . . to recognize early the nature of pathological cases and send for the timely help of the physician.

The Playfair School offered diplomas in midwifery as well as certificates in obstetric nursing to those women who did not wish to qualify fully as midwives.[26]

The 1899 annual announcement of the Playfair School listed eleven faculty members, ten of whom held the M.D. degree and six of whom were women. There were two major admission requirements. First, the prospective midwife had to present a certificate of good moral character, signed by either a physician or a minister. Second, she had to show evidence of an ability to read and write in English or German. The course consisted of two terms, each five months in length. Instruction was given in both English and German. Lectures, demonstrations, and recitations were scheduled daily from 9:00 A.M. to noon. Clinical work was conducted at the Playfair Lying-in Hospital Dispensary. Midwives who had graduated from other schools or who had been in practice for at least three years could, if they passed an entrance examination, qualify for graduation at the end of one term. The cost of the complete ten-month course was $110. In order to graduate, the student had to attend at least 80 percent of all the lectures, pass all examinations given by the various branches of the school, and show satisfactory evidence of having attended twelve cases of labor. Because of the "high grade requirements" of the Playfair School, the Illinois State Board of Health exempted its graduates from any additional state examinations exacted of midwives.[27]

A third school for midwives whose diplomas were of real value was the St. Louis College of Midwifery. One of its founders, Dr. A. A. Henske, was so concerned about improving the quality of midwife education that he also established a monthly journal, the *American Midwife*, which appeared between November 1895 and October 1896. The college offered a five-month course of instruction in English and German. Six of the eight faculty members were men with the M.D. and/or Ph.D. degrees. The two women on the faculty, Katharina Zratz and Annie J. Byrns, were trained midwives.[28]

Unfortunately, information about all three of these schools is incomplete and of uneven quality. They were evidently not important enough to merit inclusion among the topics for discussion usually found in the standard medical journals at the turn of the twentieth century. On those very rare occasions when schools for midwives were discussed, vague, condemnatory phrases were employed. Schools were not specifically identified by name. They were generally characterized as "frauds of the worst description."[29] The pioneering studies of the midwife situation in New York City and Chicago, published respectively in 1907 and 1908, made no specific mention of either the College of Midwifery of New York City or the Playfair School of Midwifery. Possibly, the two schools were no longer in existence or else they were judged to be diploma mills. Moreover, the number of students who enrolled in the three schools represented only a tiny minority of the women who acted as midwives at the turn of the century.[30]

Very few printed materials were published expressly for American midwives during the late nineteenth and early twentieth centuries. A variety of maternity and mother's manuals appeared during this period, but they were written for the educated, middle- and upper-class woman. For example, one of the most popular works of this type was Frederick Hollick's, *The Matron's Manual of Midwifery and the Diseases of Women During Pregnancy and in Child Bed.* When first published in 1848, Hollick proudly announced that it was "the first popular, and yet strictly *scientific* and *practical* book on Midwifery every published. . . ." The author made it clear that the object of the book was "not to make *every* woman a professional midwife . . . but simply to explain to her the nature and manner of child-birth, and the means by which she is to be assisted." He hoped the book would enable women to understand "everything connected with their own systems, and of the wonderful phenomena in which they play so important a part." *The Matron's Manual of Midwifery* was over 450 pages in length, and it covered virtually every aspect of pregnancy and the puerperium from the signs of pregnancy to the diseases of women in childbed. The author endorsed the use of chloroform to prevent pain, while he cautioned against the frequent employment of the forceps. He also described the way in which the male physician could properly and delicately perform a vaginal examination. The book was so popular that it was reprinted in Hollick's mammoth work, *The Origin of Life and Process of Reproduction in Plants and Animals, with the Anatomy and Physiology of the Human Generative System, Male and Female, and the Causes, Prevention and Cure of the Special Diseases to Which It is Liable.* In the preface of this work, Hollick reiterated that *The Matron's Manual of Midwifery* was published for the "private and popular use" of married women.[31]

Numerous other maternity manuals were published at this time. These books were also directed toward an audience of middle- and upper-class women. They were not written for the immigrant or black midwife. Significantly, most books of this type omitted any mention of the role of the midwife in the birth process. They assumed that both a physician and monthly nurse would be in attendance. Even Ferdinand Herb's, *Beauty and Motherhood* (1915), which was advertised as "a great book for midwives," contained little relevant information. Rather, Herb described how women could maintain their beauty both during and after pregnancy.[32]

The growing number of obstetric textbooks for students and practitioners that were published around the turn of the twentieth century were also unsuitable for midwives. These works were often quite lengthy and written in highly technical language that was difficult for the average person, untrained in the medical sciences, to understand. A great deal of attention was usually devoted to complicated and controversial topics, such as operative obstetrics and anesthesia in childbirth, that had little to do with the type of services provided by midwives.[33]

Some British manuals for midwives were also available to American women. However, midwives in the United States were discouraged from reading the British works because they were considered to be too difficult for them to understand. One American reviewer of Henry Fly Smith's *The Handbook for Midwives,* published in London in 1873, argued that it was "too elaborate for the understanding of the majority of the female nurses [in the United States] who have only to carry out the directions of the attending physician, and do not need to be acquainted with the anatomical, physiological, and pathological details of parturition."[34]

With the passage of the British Midwives Act in 1902, a variety of manuals were published in Great Britain for the purpose of preparing prospective midwives for the examination given by the Central Midwives Board. Several of these works, including Comyns Berkeley, *A Handbook for Midwives and Maternity Nurses* (1909) and A. B. Calder, *Lectures on Midwifery for Midwives* (1905), were also published in the United States. These lengthy, relatively sophisticated books were probably unintelligible to most immigrant and black midwives. As late as 1925, the British manuals were deemed inappropriate for study by the "typical rural midwife" in the United States because they might prove dangerous in the hands of the average American midwife who was "not to be trusted with a . . . bag equipped with needles, hypodermic syringes, ergot, and pituitrin. . . ."[35]

The aforementioned *American Midwife*, which was printed in both German and English, was probably the only turn-of-the-century journal published expressly for American midwives. Its founder, Dr. A. A. Henske, and many of the contributing authors were members of the faculty of the St. Louis College of Midwifery. Although only twelve issues were published, the notices that appeared within its pages indicate that at least some of its readers felt that the *American Midwife* was much-needed and greatly appreciated its existence. Congratulatory letters from midwives in such diverse locations as St. Louis, Missouri, Bensenville, Illinois, and San Francisco, California, were published. Edna L. Bartells of Bensenville wrote that "the midwife ought to have something to read just as well as the doctor, so as to remind her of her duties to her calling. As a rule she does not read any journal or book, but even forgets what she has learned." One early subscriber, Emma E. Peters, urged other midwives to send in their subscription fee of $1 for "midwives are never through learning." Medical practitioners also congratulated the editors for their endeavors. In assessing the success of the periodical, the editors reported in January 1896 that "our list of subscribers increases daily; in fact, far beyond our expectations. There is no city in this country which has not added a number of names to it." They concluded that the *American Midwife* "should be the journal that will furnish the midwife with well written articles, treating on different subjects of her science, and will keep her well advised of all the latest advances and of all important discoveries in the different branches of obstetrics."[36]

Most of the articles that were published in the *American Midwife*

were written by physicians. They dealt with a variety of topics relating to pregnancy and the puerperium including placenta praevia,
the prolapsed uterus, aseptic midwifery, abnormal uterine pains
during labor, resuscitation of the apparently stillborn infant, the
cesarean section, and anesthesia in childbirth. Occasionally, midwives wrote about their own particular experiences. Lillian V. Young,
a student at the St. Louis College of Midwifery, discussed the importance of clinical training. She stated that her first childbirth
case was normal, but that she considered it an "ordeal" because of
her lack of clinical experience. Young did not hold the St. Louis
College of Midwifery responsible for her predicament. She maintained that this was a problem common to midwifery colleges
throughout the United States. Annie J. Byrns, a trained midwife
and a faculty member at the St. Louis College of Midwifery, related
how she stopped the hemorrhaging of one patient by using a foun-
tain syringe to inject "three quarts of hot water and one pint of
strong vinegar into the vagina."[37]

Significantly, Byrns also wrote an article in which she was highly
critical of those physicians who called for the elimination of midwives on account of their alleged ignorance relating to matters of
childbirth. Byrns argued that "the United States can boast of midwives who not only wash their hands with soap, but scrub them to
their elbows, clean their finger nails, and then use antiseptic solution." She pointed out that thousands of concerned midwives read
the *American Midwife* and that midwives from St. Louis had organized the Scientific Association of Midwives for the purpose of
keeping "themselves abreast with the times." Byrns also stated that
midwives should not be denounced for their lack of knowledge.
She believed the real culprits were "the schools and State Boards of
Health" who continued to turn out "incompetent graduates and
licentiates." Thus, she maintained that better training programs
and more rigid examinations would help bring about the establishment of "a good class of midwives."[38]

When the last issue of the *American Midwife* appeared, the editors
provided no explanation for its cessation. Certainly, the claim that
its subscribers came from every city in the United States was an
exaggeration. The scant number of issues of this journal that have
survived to the present probably suggests that the subscription

roster was not very large and that women in every city in the United States did not subscribe to it.[39] Nevertheless, the significance of the *American Midwife* must not be underestimated. The fact that Henske and the other faculty members at the St. Louis College of Midwifery believed that American midwives would support the journal is important. Apparently, there were conscientious midwives in St. Louis and other areas of the United States at the turn of the century who were very concerned about improving their knowledge of pregnancy and parturition and keeping abreast of the major midwifery developments. For such women, the only publication they could turn to was the *American Midwife*. For a brief period, American midwives had a journal in which they could relate their experiences and even reply to the criticisms of those physicians who maintained that they were "dirty and ignorant." After it ceased publication, over two decades elapsed before another journal for American midwives was established.

Although it is not possible to create an exact replica of the American midwife at the turn of the twentieth century, it has been possible, through the examination of a variety of sources, to envisage what she may have been like. She would, most likely, have been a married woman who had borne several children and who had received her first training from her mother or some other older woman. Whether she was an immigrant midwife living in the urban Northeast or a black "granny" living in the rural South, she would have had little, if any, formal midwifery training. Only a very small percentage of the total number of midwives were trained at quality schools, such as the Playfair School of Midwifery in Chicago. The smattering of education that she received focused on how to manage normal confinements and which symptoms merited the calling-in of a physician. Her lack of formal training and her unfamiliarity with modern obstetric techniques meant that she usually let nature take its course. Her practice was frequently limited to friends and relatives. Not surprisingly, therefore, the income she derived from her work was quite small. The average fee charged by the midwife was less than one-half that of the general practitioner. Moreover, arrangements were often made for payment in kind. In addition, she also performed a variety of housewifely functions which were not required of a doctor. She had only limited contact with other midwives and, for the most part, went about her work unobtrusively. Occasionally, individuals, such as Dr. A. A. Henske, attempted to establish training and regulatory programs for midwives. The medical profession and the public provided little support for such programs. Indeed, in 1900 the midwife appeared to be a forgotten issue.

By 1910, however, physicians, public health advocates, and to a lesser extent the general public were embroiled in a fierce debate over the midwife question. The apathy of 1900 had been shattered by a variety of unforeseen developments and events. Individuals who ten years earlier had had no opinion about the midwife were writing and speaking to great effect. The present and future existence of the midwife was now at stake.

NOTES

1. The Bureau of the Census did not begin publishing statistical information with regard to the attendant at birth until 1937. *Vital Statistics of the United States*, 1937-1970 (Washington, D.C.), annual volumes. Most turn-of-the-century observers estimated that at least 50 percent of all births were attended by midwives. See, for example, Thomas Darlington, "The Present Status of the Midwife," *American Journal of Obstetrics and the Diseases of Women and Children*, 63 (1911), 870; Grace Abbott, "The Midwife in Chicago," *American Journal of Sociology*, 20 (March 1915), 684.

2. Helen M. Dart, *Maternity and Child Care in Selected Rural Areas of Mississippi*, United States Department of Labor, Children's Bureau Publication, No. 88 (Washington, D.C., 1921), p. 27. "The Midwives of Chicago," *Journal of the American Medical Association*, 50 (April 1908), 1346; Viola I. Paradise, *Maternity Care and the Welfare of Young Children in a Homesteading County in Montana*, United States Department of Labor, Children's Bureau Publication, No. 34 (Washington, D.C., 1919), pp. 30-32; Elizabeth Moore, *Maternity and Infant Care in a Rural County in Kansas*, United States Department of Labor, Children's Bureau Publication, No. 26 (Washington, D.C., 1917), pp. 22-23.

3. Statistics on hospital and home deliveries are sketchy for the years prior to 1940. One of the first attempts to collect information of this type occurred in 1916 when the Department of Health of New York City reported that 19.1 percent of all births in the borough of Manhattan took place in hospitals. Lee W. Thomas, "The Supervision of Midwives in New York City," *Monthly Bulletin*, Department of Health, City of New York, 9 (May 1919), 117. A report issued by the United States Children's Bureau

for the year 1921 pointed out that hospital confinements occurred much more frequently in cities than in rural areas. For example, "of the births in Baltimore, 18.7 percent occurred in hospitals, as compared with only 2.6 percent of the births in Maryland outside of Baltimore." Robert M. Woodbury, *Maternal Mortality: The Risk of Death in Childbirth and From All Diseases Caused by Pregnancy and Confinement*, United States Department of Labor, Children's Bureau Publication, No. 158 (Washington, D.C., 1926), p. 54. The first national statistics on hospital deliveries appeared in 1935. In that year, a study conducted by the United States Children's Bureau reported that 36.9 percent of all births occurred in hospitals. Elizabeth Tandy, *Infant and Maternal Mortality Among Negroes*, United States Department of Labor, Children's Bureau Publication, No. 243 (Washington, D.C., 1937), p. 7.

4. George W. Kosmak, "Maternity Hospital Care for the Woman of Moderate Means," *Transactions of the American Association for the Study and Prevention of Infant Mortality*, 4 (1913), 208; Edward P. Davis, "The Need of Hospitals for Maternity Surgical Cases," *Transactions of the American Association for the Study and Prevention of Infant Mortality*, 5 (1914), 196-201.

Margaret Sanger, who served as a nurse on the Lower East Side of New York City during the early years of the twentieth century, stated in her autobiography that

few people wanted to enter hospitals; they were afraid they might be 'practiced' upon, and consented to go only in desperate emergencies. Sentiment was especially vehement in the matter of having babies. A woman's own bedroom, no matter how inconveniently arranged, was the usual place for her lying-in.

Although Sanger did not act in the official capacity of a midwife, she admitted that on many occasions she "had to perform the delivery by myself," because labor terminated before the doctor arrived. Margaret Sanger, *An Autobiography* (New York, 1971; reprint of 1938 edition), pp. 55, 86.

5. Estelle B. Hunter, *Infant Mortality: Results of a Field Study in Waterbury, Connecticut. Based on Births in One Year*, United States Department of Labor, Children's Bureau Publication, No. 29 (Washington, D.C., 1918), p. 45; Dart, *Maternity and Child Care*, pp. 27-32.

6. S. Josephine Baker, "Discussion," *Transactions of the American Association for the Study and Prevention of Infant Mortality*, 3 (1912), 252; "Report of the Midwife Survey in Texas," (mimeographed, Texas State Board of Health, 1924), 3.

7. Rosemary Stevens, *American Medicine and the Public Interest* (New Haven, Conn., 1971), p. 99; Taliaferro Clark, "Training of Midwives," *Chicago Medical Recorder*, 46 (1924), 297-304.

Both supporters and critics of the American midwife agreed that European midwives were much better trained and supervised than their counterparts in the United States. S. Josephine Baker, an ardent defender of the early twentieth-century American midwife, presented a paper to the 1911 meeting of the American Association for the Study and Prevention of Infant Mortality in which she summarized her research regarding the training and regulation of midwives in some half-dozen European countries. Baker maintained that "Europe has struck the keynote by not only recognizing that preliminary education and training is essential, but in most instances providing facilities for procuirng it, . . ." She also stated that "the best midwives in this country are those who have been graduated from European schools." S. Josephine Baker, "Schools for Midwives," *Transactions of the American Association for the Study and Prevention of Infant Mortality*, 2 (1911), 233-237.

At the same 1911 meeting, Arthur B. Emmons and James L. Huntington, two vocal anti-midwife physicians, pointed out that the German midwife was highly trained and well supervised. Moreover, the findings of Emmons and Huntington were based, to a large extent, on firsthand observation. After witnessing the final examination of a prospective German midwife, they concluded that "we can definitely state that it is a thorough and severe test of the candidate's knowledge of the subject—it is one that the average graduate of an American medical school would have difficulty in passing with distinction." Arthur B. Emmons and James L. Huntington, "Has the Trained and Supervised Midwife Made Good?" *Transactions of the American Association for the Study and Prevention of Infant Mortality*, 2 (1911), 203.

8. Hunter, *Infant Mortality*, p. 45; Jessamine S. Whitney, *Infant Mortality: Results of a Field Study in New Bedford, Massachusetts. Based on Births in One Year*, United States Department of Labor, Children's Bureau Publication, No. 68 (Washington, D.C., 1920), p. 31; F. Elisabeth Crowell, "The Midwives of New York," *Charities and the Commons*, 17 (January 1907), 668.

9. H. J. Garrigues, "Midwives," *Medical News*, 72 (1898), 235; Elizabeth Shaver, "Infant Mortality and the Midwife Problem," *Louisville (Kentucky) Monthly Journal of Medicine and Surgery*, 19 (June 1912), 25.

10. "Report of the Midwife Survey in Texas," 1-3.

11. Emma Goldman briefly commented on her experiences as a turn-of-the-century midwife in New York City in her autobiography, *Living My Life*. She stated that her

profession of midwife was not very lucrative, only the poorest of the foreign element resorting to such services. Those who had risen in the scale of material Americanism lost their native diffidence together with many other original traits. Like the American women they, too, would be confined only by doctors. Midwifery offered a very limited scope; in emergencies one was compelled to call for the aid of a physician. Ten dollars was the highest fee; the majority of the women could not pay even that. But while my work held out no hope of worldly riches, it furnished an excellent field for experience. It put me into intimate contact with the very people my ideal strove to help and emancipate.

Emma Goldman, *Living My Life* (New York, 1970; reprint of 1931 edition), I, 185.

12. White House Conference on Child Health and Protection, *Obstetric Education* (New York, 1932), pp. 178-192; Louis S. Reed, *Midwives, Chiropodists, and Optometrists: Their Place in Medical Care* (Chicago, 1932), pp. 15-16.

13. See, for example, J. Clifton Edgar, "The Remedy for the Midwife Problem," *American Journal of Obstetrics and the Diseases of Women and Children*, 63 (1911), 881; Emmons and Huntington, "Has the Trained and Supervised Midwife," 207-208; W. A. Plecker, "The Midwife in Virginia," *Virginia Medical Semi-Monthly*, 18 (January 1914), 475; Charles E. Terry, "The Mother, the Midwife and the Law," *Delineator*, 92 (February 1916), 12-13.

14. Crowell, "Midwives of New York," 673; "Midwives of Chicago," 1348.

Emma Goldman discussed the frequent requests she received from poor women in New York City asking her to perform illegal abortions. Goldman stated,

Many women called me for that purpose [of performing an abortion], even going down on their knees and begging me to help them, "for the sake of the poor little ones already here." They knew some doctors and midwives did such things, but the price was beyond their means. . . . I tried to explain to them that it was not monetary considerations that held me back; it was concern for their life and health. I would relate the case of a woman killed by such an operation, and her children left motherless. But they preferred to die, they avowed; the city was then sure to take care of their orphans, and they would be better off.

Goldman, *Living*, I, 186.

15. Guy Steele, "The Midwife Problem and Its Legal Control," *Maryland Medical Journal*, 48 (January 1905), 2, 4; Helmina Jeidell and Willa M. Fricke, "The Midwives of Anne Arundel, County, Maryland," *Johns Hopkins Hospital Bulletin*, 23 (1912), 281; Marie Campbell, *Folks Do Get Born* (New York, 1946), p. 33; Carolyn C. Van Blarcom, "Midwives in America," *American Journal of Public Health*, 4 (March 1914), 198; Carolyn C. Van Blarcom, "Rat Pie: Among the Black Midwives of the South," *Harper's*, 160 (February 1930), 325.

16. Dart, *Maternity and Child Care*, p. 23; Glenn Steele, *Maternity and Infant Care in a Mountain County in Georgia*, United States Department of

Labor, Children's Bureau Publication, No. 120 (Washington, D.C., 1923), p. 17.

17. Dart, *Maternity and Child Care*, p. 22; Steele, *Maternity and Infant Care*, p. 16.

18. *Atlanta Constitution*, September 16, 1974, 6A.

19. "Midwives of Chicago," 1348-1349; Abbott, "Midwife in Chicago," 690; Crowell, "Midwives of New York," 671.

20. Crowell, "Midwives of New York," 671; "Midwives of Chicago," 1349.

21. Clark, "Training of Midwives," 297-304; Baker, "Schools for Midwives," 233-234; Arthur B. Emmons and James L. Huntington stated in 1911 that "the finely trained midwife who comes with her diploma and her sterilizer from the schools of the Old World, finding no use for either of these articles, forgets that she ever possessed them and becomes to all intents and purposes an untrained midwife." Emmons and Huntington, "Has the Trained and Supervised Midwife," 206.

22. Claire Noall, "Mormon Midwives," *Utah Historical Quarterly*, 10 (1942), 133. Noall states that the "Mother of Mormon Midwifery" was Patty Sessions. She was born in Bethel, Maine, in 1795. At the age of thirty-nine she joined the Church of Jesus Christ of Latter-day Saints. In 1836, she and her husband left Maine in order to join other groups of Mormons in the West. After living in Ohio and Illinois, they eventually settled in Utah. From 1846 to 1880, Sessions kept a diary of her experiences as a midwife and general doctor. It is located at the archives of the Latter-day Saints Church Historian's Office, Salt Lake City, Utah. (84-110)

23. *Woman's Work in the Field of Medicine* (New York, 1883), pp. 19-20, 27.

24 Ibid., pp. 8, 21-24.

25. Ibid., pp. 6-8.

26. *Playfair School of Midwifery: Annual Announcement, 1899* (Chicago, 1899), pp. 6-8.

27. Ibid., pp. 7, 13-16.

28. See the advertisements for the St. Louis College of Midwifery appearing in each issue of the *American Midwife*, 1 (1895)-2(1896).

29. C. S. Bacon, "The Midwife Question in America," *Journal of the American Medical Association*, 29 (1897), 1090.

30. Crowell, "Midwives of New York," 667-677; "Midwives of Chicago," 1346-1350.

31. Frederick Hollick, *The Matron's Manual of Midwifery and the Diseases of Women during Pregnancy and in Child Bed* (New York, 1848), pp. iii-iv, passim.; Federick Hollick, *The Origin of Life and Process of Reproduction in Plants and Animals, with the Anatomy and Physiology of the Human Generative System, Male and Female, and the Causes, Prevention and Cure of the Special Diseases to Which It is Liable* (Philadelphia, 1878), xii.

32. See Chapter 1, note 45; "Advertisement," *Topics of Interest to Midwives,* 2 (January 1918), 4; Ferdinand Herb, *Beauty and Motherhood* (Chicago, 1915), Chapter 30.

33. See, for example, Rodney Glisan, *Textbook of Modern Midwifery* (Philadelphia, 1881); Charles Jewett, *Outlines of Obstetrics: A Syllabus of Lectures Delivered at the Long Island College Hospital* (Philadelphia, 1894); J. Whitridge Williams, *Obstetrics: A Textbook for the Use of Students and Practitioners* (New York, 1903).

34. "Handbook for Midwives," *American Journal of Obstetrics and the Diseases of Women and Children,* 6 (1873-1874), 700.

35. "Reviews and Book Notes," *Public Health Nurse,* 17 (April 1925), 220-221.

36. "Letters," *American Midwife,* 1 (December 1895), 6; "Editorial," *American Midwife,* 1 (January 1896), 1.

37. "Letters," *American Midwife,* 1 (February 1896), 15; Annie J. Byrns, "From My Practices," *American Midwife,* 1 (November 1895), 5.

38. Annie J. Byrns, "Midwives," *American Midwife,* 1 (December 1895), 4-5.

39. Only three libraries in the United States possess copies of the *American Midwife.* The two most complete files of the journal are located at the library of the College of Physicians of Philadelphia and the St. Louis Society for Medical and Scientific Education.

4

Prelude to the Early Twentieth-Century Midwife Debate

During the early years of the twentieth century two major developments unfolded which caused the medical profession, public health officials, and lay people to take note of the midwife. First, physicians became increasingly concerned about medical education reform and the related issue of "overcrowding" in the profession.[1] Many physicians believed that eliminating the midwife, or at least substantially reducing her numbers, would help alleviate this dual problem.

As early as 1898, H. J. Garrigues, a New York City obstetrician, expressed concern about the "superabundance of medical men" in need of additional obstetric cases.[2] Throughout the late 1890s and well into the twentieth century, American physicans worried about the "overcrowding" of the medical profession. One doctor wrote in 1907 that "it has been estimated that it requires one thousand of the population to insure a physician a decent living, yet in these United States the average is one physician to seven hundred or eight hundred population."[3] Doctors maintained that overcrowding had resulted in a loss of their status and a diminution of their income. Not surprisingly, they began to devise plans for the purpose of limiting the number of medical practitioners.[4]

State licensing and control was one technique that was used in an effort to limit the number of physicians. State licensure programs experienced only limited success, however, because of the lack of uniform state laws and the conflicts that arose from attempts to formulate a workable system of reciprocity.[5] Much more successful in restricting the number of physicians was the movement to control medical education by limiting the number of schools and the number of graduates. Numerous articles on the need for reform in medical education appeared in the *Journal of the American Medical Association* and other medical journals of the period. The "proprietary schools" were specifically singled out for criticism because they advanced "commercialism" in medicine and encouraged "the poor and the working class to be physicians."[6]

Not satisfied with merely voicing complaints about American medical education, the American Medical Association established its influential Council on Medical Education in 1904. The council worked to improve the quality of medical education by establishing its own maximum and minimum standards for medical schools. While medical schools were not legally required to follow the guidelines established by the council, its suggestions were often followed as if they were the law. In addition, in 1906 the council began an extensive survey of medical schools throughout the United States, rating them A (acceptable), B (doubtful), and C (unacceptable). Of the 160 schools inspected in 1906-1907, only 82 were placed in the A classification. The work of the council undoubtedly contributed to the closing or merger of 29 medical schools between 1906 and 1910.[7] Of course, different groups were affected unevenly by the consolidation movement. The number of students attending homeopathic, eclectic, and other "irregular" medical schools dropped dramatically after 1900. Similarly, medical schools for women and blacks were forced to close their doors swiftly.[8]

The Council on Medical Education also secured the cooperation of the Carnegie Foundation for the Advancement of Teaching in its efforts to bring about reform in American medical education.[9] In November 1908, the Carnegie Foundation appointed Abraham Flexner to direct a study on medical education in the United States. During the next two years, Flexner and his assistants visited over 150 American medical schools in an attempt to determine the quality of education that medical students were receiving. The final report was issued in 1910, and it reaffirmed the view that the medical profession was overcrowded. The *Flexner Report* concluded that

"for twenty-five years past there has been an enormous over-pro-
duction of uneducated and ill-trained medical practitioners. Taking
the United States as a whole, physicians are four to five times as
numerous in proportion to the population as in older countries like
Germany." In order to alleviate this situation, the report recommended the reduction of the 155 medical schools in America to 31.
These 31 schools were to be strategically situated throughout the
United States. Ideally, they would be located in large cities, capable
of providing adequate hospital facilities and clinical material. Each
incoming student would be required to have a minimum of two
years of college education before beginning the four-year course of
instruction in medicine.[10]

The Carnegie Foundation's investigation of American medical
education marked the first time, an "independent educational
agency" had entered the campaign to bring about the consolidation
and elimination of medical schools. Moreover, other private groups
soon began to contribute substantial sums of money to the consolidation movement. Foundations, such as Rockefeller and Carnegie, were able "to finance the consolidation and development of . . .
chosen centers of [medical] research" at the expense of medical
colleges for women and blacks as well as those schools located in
rural areas of the United States.[11]

Once Flexner's findings were made public, other investigations
were undertaken which examined specific aspects of medical education. The field of obstetrics was closely scrutinized. Many physicians were especially distressed about the poor quality of obstetric
education and the degraded status of the obstetrician. They believed
that the midwife was at least partially responsible for their dilemma.
If obstetrics were to receive its due recognition, the midwife had to
be eliminated.[12]

The second, and equally significant, development that was responsible for the upsurge of interest in the midwife around 1910
was the revelation that the maternal and infant mortality rates in
the United States were alarmingly high. Prior to the early years of
the twentieth century, only a few large cities maintained adequate
birth and death statistics. In 1880, however, the Bureau of Census
established a death registration area. The annual collection and
publication of mortality statistics within the registration area began

in 1900. The original death registration area included only two states (Massachusetts and New Jersey). The area was gradually expanded and by 1933 it included all forty-eight states. Similarly, a birth registration area was established in 1915. It, too, was gradually expanded to include all forty-eight states by 1933.[13] Once these birth and death statistics were made public, physicians and health officials began to question the midwife's role in the birth process and to try to determine why the maternal and infant mortality rates of the United States were so high. Moreover, the recognition that many mothers and infants were needlessly dying propelled federal, state, and municipal health agencies to initiate programs that were intended to reduce these rates.[14]

New York City enacted the first large-scale program of this type.[15] The initial step was taken in 1906 when the Public Health Committee of the Association of Neighborhood Workers commissioned F. Elisabeth Crowell, a nurse, to conduct a study of the midwives of New York City. In her report, Crowell was highly critical of "the usual type of woman who follows the calling of midwife in this country. The majority of these so-called midwives are foreigners of a low grade—ignorant, untrained women who find in the natural needs and life-long prejudice of the parturient woman a lucrative means of livelihood."[16]

Crowell's scathing indictment of midwives prompted the city to revise its laws pertaining to their regulation. Prior to 1907, the woman who wished to register as a midwife merely had to appear in person at the office of the Registrar of Records and present a certificate, signed by two physicians, attesting that she was experienced in midwifery and of good moral character. The new law passed by New York City on June 6, 1907, tightened the rules and regulations governing the midwife and specifically excluded her from "the assisting of child-birth by any artificial, forcible or mechanical means, nor the performance of version, nor the removal of adherent placenta, nor the administering, prescribing, advising, or employing in child-birth of any drug other than a disinfectant."[17]

The following year the Bureau of Child Hygiene of the Department of Health of the City of New York was created. It was the first municipal bureau in the United States established for the purpose of improving the health of infants and children. Eventually, similar city and state bureaus were modeled after it. The director of the bureau, Dr. S. Josephine Baker, served more than twenty-five years with the Department of Health and was a key figure in the movement to establish a program for the training and regulation of midwives. She also sought to bring about the reduction of the infant and maternal mortality rates of New York City by providing prenatal instruction for mothers, establishing baby health stations and Little Mother Leagues, campaigning for pure milk, and distributing educational materials to expectant mothers.[18]

New York City further demonstrated its leadership in the field of midwife training and control by establishing the first municipally sponsored school for midwives in 1911. It was a branch of Bellevue Hospital and was called the Bellevue School for Midwives. The original course of instruction was six months in length, but it was soon expanded to cover eight months. Both practical and theoretical instruction was given by physicians and nurses. The training program included instruction in prenatal and postpartum care, the procedures to be followed during cases of normal labor, infant feeding, care of the infant, and the essential housewifely duties to be performed by the midwife. Most of the students were of Italian, German, Polish, or Hungarian descent. There were no special admission requirements other than that the prospective midwife be able to read and write and be of good moral character. There was no charge for the course. Most reports issued by physicians and public health officials during the second decade of the twentieth century agreed that the Bellevue School for Midwives was the *only* institution in the United States that provided an adequate education for midwives. One early report, published by the Department of Health, described the students as "intelligent, earnest women with sufficient education to grasp the principles of normal obstetrics, asepsis, and to recognize abnormalities. . . ." Interestingly, nurses were not allowed admission to the Bellevue School for Midwives because it did "not have accommodations suitable" for them. The enrollment figures for the years 1913-1917 were as follows: 1913, 22; 1914, 40; 1915, 61; 1916, 37; 1917, 50.[19]

Four years after the establishment of the school, the regulations governing the practices of midwives in New York City were modified so that only those women who had graduated from a recognized school of midwifery could qualify for a license. The only school in the United States recognized by the Bureau of Child Hygiene was the one at Bellevue Hospital. The school remained in existence until 1935, when a lack of students forced it to close its doors.[20]

The United States Children's Bureau, established in 1912 within the United States Department of Labor, was another organization that worked to reduce infant and maternal mortality rates in the United States. Around 1903, a variety of social workers, most notably Lillian Wald and Florence Kelley of the Henry Street Settlement House in New York City, began pushing for the creation of a federally sponsored children's bureau. Not until the 1909 White House Conference on Children recommended that such a bureau be established were the necessary preparations for its organization begun. One of the first and most important projects undertaken by the bureau's chief, Julia C. Lathrop, was an ongoing investigation of the maternal and infant care provided in various rural and urban localities throughout the United States.[21]

In a 1917 landmark study, *Maternal Mortality From All Conditions Connected With Childbirth in the United States and Certain Other Countries*, the bureau reported that "childbirth caused more deaths among women fifteen to forty-four years old than any disease except tuberculosis." Moreover, the statistics available for the years 1890-1913 indicated no apparent decrease in the maternal death rate. For the expanding death registration area of the United States for the years 1890 to 1913, the maternal death rate per 100,000 population was 15.3 in 1890, 13 in 1902, and 15.8 in 1913. Perhaps the most alarming statistics included in the 1917 study were those that compared the maternal mortality rate of the United States with fifteen foreign countries. Only two of fifteen countries investigated had maternal mortality rates higher than the United States for the period 1900 to 1910.[22]

The statistics relating to infant mortality were just as disturbing as the maternal mortality figures.[23] The infant mortality statistics for the death registration area of the United States in 1910 was 124 deaths per 1,000 live births. Statistics in certain localities were much higher than the national average. The infant mortality rate of Manchester, New Hampshire, as an example, was 165 deaths per 1,000 live births in 1913. The 1913 figure for Waterbury, Connecticut, was 174.1. Primarily because of the efforts of the Children's Bureau, the infant mortality rate for the birth registration area of the United States was reduced to 101 by 1916. This figure was still substantially higher than was reported by some of the major European countries for the same period. For example, in 1916 the infant mortality rate for the Netherlands was 85, while Switzerland reported a rate of 78 and Norway, 64. Moreover, New Zealand's infant mortality rate was 51—only one-half that of the United States.[24]

Following the example of New York City and with the aid of the federal Children's Bureau, cities and states throughout the United States began to establish special bureaus to deal specifically with improving the health of their infants and children. Most of the bureaus were created between 1919 and 1921. By 1924, all forty-eight states had established a bureau of child hygiene or its equivalent. These bureaus issued reports on numerous child-related topics including the pure milk movement, the prevention of ophthalmia neonatorum, child labor legislation, adequate prenatal care for all mothers, and the training and regulation of midwives.[25]

Before the advent of such bureaus, most state boards of health did not even know how many midwives were practicing within their boundaries. When S. Josephine Baker sent out a midwife questionnaire to all the state boards of health in 1911, she received thirty-five incomplete sets of answers. Only six states could report the number of midwives in practice, and only one had a record of the number of births reported by them. Thirteen states indicated that they had laws regulating the practice of midwives, but the enforcement of the laws was usually left up to the local authorities. On some occasions, the city or town law differed from the state law. Schools for midwives were reported to exist in New Jersey, New York, Ohio, Utah, and Wisconsin. Except for the Bellevue School for Midwives in New York City, the curricula of the schools were unknown and state supervision was minimal or nonexistent.[26]

Once bureaus of child hygiene were established, several northern localities, most notably Connecticut, New Jersey, and New York City, began conducting investigations on the midwife situation. They sponsored numerous educational programs for midwives, such as short (ten-week) courses on midwifery. They held periodic institutes in which physicians and trained midwives spoke about various topics relating to pregnancy and parturition. The bureaus of child hygiene also encouraged midwives to form their own midwife clubs where they could share their midwifery experiences. In several instances, state midwifery supervisors were appointed for the purpose of coordinating the educational programs and the regulation of midwives.[27]

By the early and mid-1920s, the bureaus of child hygiene of many southern states were also taking an active interest in their midwives. Public health nurses were appointed to travel throughout the rural areas of the South in order to help the "grannies" form midwife clubs. These nurses visited the homes of the "grannies," inspected their bags, and impressed upon them the necessity of asepsis during parturition. Manuals for midwives were published and short midwifery courses were also offered. Significant investigations of the midwife situation, such as the 1924 "Report on the Midwife Survey in Texas," were conducted.[28]

Many cities and states also began to enact new laws or revise already existing laws pertaining to midwives. New York City's 1915 statute requiring the licensed midwife to be a graduate of a recognized school of midwifery was much more stringent than most of the laws that were passed. Generally, the laws were concerned with defining the midwife's activities and preventing her from attending abnormal births. She was often prohibited from using drugs, instruments, or performing vaginal examinations. The law frequently stipulated that she register all births and report any cases of ophthalmia neonatorum among the babies that she delivered. Another specification usually written into the law was that the midwife must apply silver nitrate to the newborn infant's eyes as an ophthalmia prophylaxis.[29]

Not all states attempted to regulate the practices of the midwife. Maine, for example, enacted no special midwifery legislation between 1900 and 1930. The only legal recognition of the Maine midwife occurred with the passage of the 1895 Medical Practice Act, which exempted her from its provisions because she "lay[s] no claim to the title of physician or doctor." The *Bulletins* issued by the Maine State Board of Health for the years 1905-1922 also included very little information about the midwife. Although there were some published reports that discussed the high infant mortality rates of various Maine towns and cities, these deaths were usually attributed to the impure milk supply rather than to the midwife.[30]

Massachusetts was the only state during the 1900-1930 period that actually outlawed the midwife. The 1901 Medical Practice Act of Massachusetts, which set forth the legal requirements for the practice of medicine, listed obstetrics as a major branch of medicine. Unlike many other states that enacted similar legislation, however, Massachusetts did not distinguish the work of the midwife from that of the medical practitioner. This meant that Massachusetts midwives could not legally attend births unless they could qualify to practice medicine as defined by the 1901 Medical Practice Act. In the same year, a law was passed which required midwives to register any births that they attended.[31] Thus, the Massachusetts legislature placed the midwife in the anomalous position of making her practice illegal while requiring her to register the births she attended. A decision by the Massachusetts Superior Court in 1907 upheld the constitutionality of the 1901 Medical Practice Act and convicted Hanna Porn, a trained and practicing midwife, of violating its provisions. Interestingly, the presiding judge was basically sympathetic to Porn's predicament. In his concluding remarks, Judge J. Rugg pointed out that it was certainly

within the power of the Legislature to separate by a line of statutory demarcation the work of the midwife from that of the practitioner in medicine. . . . The statute now under consideration does not make such a separation. . . . Whatever hardships there may be as shown by the agreed facts, comes from the scope of the statute.[32]

The only attempt to provide special legislation for Massachusetts midwives occurred in 1913 when Representative Lawrence S. Perry introduced a bill which required all midwives to register with the city or town clerk where they lived. Support for the bill was so meager that Perry withdrew it from the docket, and it never came up for a vote.[33]

No two states provided for their midwives in exactly the same way. The laws regulating midwives varied from state to state and the forty-eight separate bureaus of child hygiene worked at cross-purposes on a number of occasions. Some state and city health officials, such as S. Josephine Baker, director of the Bureau of Child Hygiene of New York City and Julius Levy, director of the New Jersey Bureau of Child Hygiene, were staunch supporters of the trained and regulated midwife. They believed that she deserved a permanent place within the medical hierarchy of the United States. Others, such as S. W. Newmayer, head of the Division of Child Hygiene for Philadelphia, felt that the midwife was a "useless institution," but that regulatory laws were necessary until every woman could be assured of receiving competent, professional medical care. Health officials in several southern states, including Alabama, Mississippi, and Virginia, also hoped that the midwife could be ultimately eliminated. The Division of Hygiene for Massachusetts probably had the most negative attitude toward the midwife of any state department of health. In 1915, the year the division was created, it called for the elimination of the midwife.[34]

Numerous other groups, in addition to the federal Children's Bureau and the state and city bureaus of child hygiene, were also interested in the midwife question. The most significant private organization concerned with the role played by the midwife in the birth process was the American Association for the Study and Prevention of Infant Mortality (AASPIM). It was founded in 1910 by a group of physicians and public health officials who were deeply disturbed about the infant mortality rate in the United States. During its first ten years of existence, the AASPIM conducted numerous investigations and its members engaged in lengthy debates about the midwife.[35] The New York Committee for the Prevention of Blindness, the Maryland Society for the Prevention of Blindness, and the Babies Milk Fund Association were a few of the other organizations that examined the midwife question during the second two decades of the twentieth century.

At the same time, numerous articles on the "midwife problem" appeared in most of the major American medical journals. Between 1910 and 1920, the future of the midwife was fiercely debated within the pages of these publications. To a lesser extent, articles on the midwife were also published in many of the popular magazines of the period. A careful analysis of the content of these articles, as well as the reports and bulletins that were issued by the Children's Bureau, the state bureaus of child hygiene, the American Association for the

Study and Prevention of Infant Mortality and other groups, helps to explain why the ranks of the midwives were decimated between 1900 and 1930. During that thirty-year period, the percentage of midwife-attended births declined from 50 to 15 percent.[36] The next two chapters will examine this decline.

NOTES

1. Of course, physicians had recognized the need for medical education reform long before the beginnings of the twentieth century. The American Medical Association, founded in 1847, had as one of its initial purposes the improvement of the quality of medical education. This same purpose was a reason for the development of state licensure laws during the last quarter of the nineteenth century. Nevertheless, the drive for medical education reform was a special and distinguishing feature of the 1890-1920 era. James G. Burrow, *AMA: Voice of American Medicine* (Baltimore, 1963), pp. 5-10; William G. Rothstein, *American Physicians in the Nineteenth Century: From Sects to Science* (Baltimore, 1972), p. 115; Robert P. Hudson, "Abraham Flexner in Perspective: American Medical Education, 1865-1910," *Bulletin of the History of Medicine,* 46 (December 1972), 545-561; Gerald E. Markowitz and David Karl Rosner, "Doctors in Crisis: A Study of the Use of Medical Education Reform to Establish Modern Professional Elitism in Medicine," *American Quarterly,* 25 (March 1973), 83-107; Rosemary Stevens, *American Medicine and the Public Interest* (New Haven, Conn., 1971), Chapter 3.

2. H. J. Garrigues, "Midwives," *Medical News,* 72 (1898), 233, 235.

3. C. L. Girard, "A Comparison of the Old-time and Modern Physician," *Journal of Michigan Medical Society,* 6 (March 1907), 107. Quoted in Markowitz and Rosner, "Doctors in Crisis," 89.

4. The most thorough examination of physicians' attitudes about overcrowding during the 1890-1910 period can be found in Markowitz and Rosner, "Doctors in Crisis," 87-97. See also Stevens, *American Medicine,* Chapter 3. Stevens states that the "reform movement was partly educational, partly restrictionist, having as its goal both more highly trained and fewer physicians." (55)

5. Stevens, *American Medicine,* pp. 61-63.

6. Markowitz and Rosner, "Doctors in Crisis," 89, 95.

7. Stevens, *American Medicine,* pp. 64-66; Hudson, "Abraham Flexner," 556.

8. Markowitz and Rosner, "Doctors in Crisis," 96-97.

9. Hudson, "Abraham Flexner," 556; D. B. Munger, "Robert Brookings and the Flexner Report," *Journal of the History of Medicine*, 23 (October 1968), 356-357.

10. Abraham Flexner, *Medical Education in the United States and Canada: A Report to the Carnegie Foundation for the Advancement of Teaching* (Boston, 1910), pp. viii, x, 26, 57, 143, 154.

11. Markowitz and Rosner, "Doctors in Crisis," 101, 102.

12. See, for example, Charles E. Ziegler, "The Elimination of the Midwife," *Transactions of the American Association for the Study and Prevention of Infant Mortality*, 3 (1912), 222-223, 258.

13. United States Bureau of the Census, *Historical Statistics of the United States, Colonial Times to 1957* (Washington, D.C., 1960), p. 18.

14. During the second half of the nineteenth century, a few physicians and lay people began to express alarm about the high infant mortality rate in the United States. By the 1880s and 1890s, concerned individuals were centering their attention around the question of infant feeding, especially the problems arising from an impure milk supply, and its relationship to the high infant mortality rate in the United States. Not until the early decades of the twentieth century, however, did a national campaign aimed at reducing infant and maternal mortality get underway. Moreover, by the early decades of the twentieth century, physicians and public health officials had recognized that a variety of factors contributed to these high death rates, including an impure milk and water supply, inadequate prenatal care, uneducated mothers, and the quality of care provided by the attendant at birth. John B. Blake, "Origins of Maternal and Child Health Programs" (mimeographed, Yale University School of Medicine, 1953), 11-42; G. F. McCleary, *The Early History of the Infant Welfare Movement* (London, 1933), Chapter IV; Grace L. Meigs, "Other Factors in Infant Mortality than the Milk and Their Control," *American Journal of Public Health*, 6 (1916), 847.

15. Blake, "Origins of Maternal," 32.

16. F. Elisabeth Crowell, "The Midwives of New York," *Charities and the Commons*, 17 (January 1907), 668.

17. "Supervision of Midwives in New York City," *Weekly Bulletin*, Department of Health, City of New York, 10 (May 1921), 154; *Regulations Governing the Practice of Midwifery in the City of New York* (New York City Department of Health, 1918), p. 3.

18. S. Josephine Baker, *Fighting for Life* (New York, 1939), pp. 111-146.

19. Lee W. Thomas, "The Supervision of Midwives in New York City," *Monthly Bulletin*, Department of Health, City of New York, 9 (May 1919), 118. Information on the origins and the early history of the Bellevue School

for Midwives is also included in the following works: S. Josephine Baker, *Child Hygiene* (New York, 1925), pp. 118-119; S. Josephine Baker, "Schools for Midwives," *American Journal of Obstetrics and the Diseases of Women and Children,* 65 (1912), 263-266; Hazel Wedgewood, "Midwifery in Massachusetts," *Commonhealth,* 8 (March-April 1921), 81-83.

20. "Supervision of Midwives in New York City," 154; George W. Kosmak, "The Midwife," *Briefs,* 8 (1944), 25.

21. Dorothy E. Bradbury, *Five Decades of Action for Children: A History of the Children's Bureau,* United States Department of Health, Education and Welfare, Children's Bureau Publication, No. 358 (Washington, D.C., 1962), pp. 1-19; Leona Baumgartner, "The American Pattern for Child Health," *Briefs,* 14 (February 1950), 4; Nancy Pottisham Weiss, "Save the Children: A History of the Children's Bureau, 1903-1918" (unpublished Ph.D. dissertation, University of California, Los Angeles, 1974), pp. 48-119. Weiss maintains that "Lathrop deliberately chose infancy as the least problematic subject of her first year's topic. To reduce controversy to a minimum, she spoke of the infant mortality investigations as 'baby saving' campaigns." (185-186)

22. Grace L. Meigs, *Maternal Mortality From All Conditions Connected With Childbirth in the United States and Certain Other Countries,* United States Department of Labor, Children's Bureau Publication, No. 19 (Washington, D.C., 1917), pp. 7, 17.

The countries with maternal death rates lower than the United States for the years 1900-1910 were as follows: Sweden (6.0); Norway (8.1); Italy (8.9); France (10.3); Prussia (10.4); England and Wales (11.1); New Zealand (12.4); Ireland (12.9); Hungary (13.3); Japan (13.3); Australia (14.1); Belgium (14.8); Scotland (14.8). The two countries with maternal mortality rates higher than the United States were Switzerland (15.2) and Spain (19.6). Ibid., p. 56.

23. Infant mortality is defined as any death that occurs during the first twelve months of life. A 1919 study conducted by the Children's Bureau reported that "two-fifths of all the infants dying the first year of life die during the first three weeks after birth." These early infant deaths were attributed to lack of adequate prenatal care and unskilled assistance during parturition and the puerperium. *Save the Youngest: Seven Charts on Maternal and Infant Mortality, with Explanatory Comment,* United States Department of Labor, Children's Bureau Publication, No. 61 (Washington, D.C., [1919]), p. 7.

24. Bradbury, *Five Decades,* p. 6; Beatrice Sheets Duncan and Emma Duke, *Infant Mortality: Results of a Field Study in Manchester, New Hampshire. Based on Births in One Year,* United States Department of Labor,

Children's Bureau Publication, No. 20 (Washington, D.C., 1917), p. 117; Estelle B. Hunter, *Infant Mortality: Results of a Field Study in Waterbury, Connecticut. Based on Births in One Year,* United States Department of Labor, Children's Bureau Publication, No. 29 (Washington, D.C., 1918), p. 17; Anna Rochester, *Infant Mortality: Results of a Field Study in Baltimore, Maryland. Based on Births in One Year,* United States Department of Labor, Children's Bureau Publication, No. 119 (Washington, D.C., 1923), p. 223.

25. Baker, *Child Hygiene,* pp. 481-484; Mary Evelyn Leith, "The Development of Midwife Education in South Carolina, 1919-1946" (unpublished M.A. thesis, Yale University, 1948), pp. 1-5.

The mounting interest in reducing the maternal and infant mortality rates in the United States during the early decades of the twentieth century should be seen as part of the larger effort by progressive reformers to protect the children of America. Robert H. Wiebe, for example, has argued that the central theme of humanitarian progressivism was the child, for "he united the campaigns for health, education, and richer city environment, and he dominated much of the interest in labor legislation." Robert H. Wiebe, *The Search for Order, 1877-1920* (New York, 1967), p. 169. Most historians, however, have failed to recognize that the endeavors of individuals, such as Baker, Kelley, Lathrop, and Wald, to reduce the maternal and infant mortality rates were part of this larger effort. For example, Robert H. Bremner and Robert H. Wiebe, focus almost exclusively on the efforts of reformers to enact child labor legislation. Robert H. Bremner, *From the Depths: The Discovery of Poverty in the United States* (New York, 1956), pp. 212-229; Wiebe, *Search,* pp. 111, 199, 220. A partial corrective to this view can be found in Weiss, "Save the Children," pp. 8-47, 120-171.

26. Baker, "Schools for Midwives," 262.

27. "Memorandum Re: Control and Practice of Midwifery in New York City" (mimeographed, New York City Bureau of Municipal Research, 1915); *Forty-Ninth Annual Report,* New Jersey State Department of Health (1926), pp. 100-102; Julius Levy, "The Maternal and Infant Mortality in Midwifery Practice in Newark, New Jersey," *American Journal of Obstetrics and the Diseases of Women and Children,* 77 (1918), 41-53; S. W. Newmayer, "The Status of Midwifery in Pennsylvania and a Study of the Midwives of Philadelphia," *Monthly Cyclopedia and Medical Bulletin,* 4 (1911), 712-719.

28. See, for example, Jessie L. Marriner, *Midwifery in Alabama* (Alabama State Board of Health, [1925]); "Georgia Midwife Plan," (mimeographed, Georgia Department of Public Health, Miscellaneous Files, Box 1, [193?]); *Report,* Board of Health of Mississippi (1919-1921), pp. 178, 197-

198; *Manual for Midwives* (Mississippi State Board of Health, 1927); *Lessons for Midwives* (Georgia State Board of Health, Box 1 [1922]); "Report of the Midwife Survey in Texas" (mimeographed, Texas State Board of Health, 1924).

29. J. A. Foote, "Legislative Measures Against Maternal and Infant Mortality," *American Journal of Obstetrics and the Diseases of Women and Children*, 80 (1919), 534-551; Robert M. Woodbury, *Maternal Mortality: The Risk of Death in Childbirth and From All Diseases Caused by Pregnancy and Confinement*, United States Department of Labor, Children's Bureau Publication, No. 158 (Washington, D.C., 1926), pp. 132-139.

30. Chapter 180, Section 10, *Acts and Resolves of the Sixty-Seventh Legislature of the State of Maine*, 1895; "Public Health Administration in Lewiston and Auburn," *Bulletin*, Maine State Department of Health, 1 (November 1918), 158; "Public Health Administration in Bangor and Bath," *Bulletin*, Maine State Department of Health, 2 (July 1919), 141-142, 147.

31. Chapter 76, Section 8, *Revised Laws of the Commonwealth of Massachusetts*, 1901; Chapter 29, Section 3, *Revised Laws of the Commonwealth of Massachusetts*, 1901.

32. *Commonwealth* v. *Hanna Porn*, *Massachusetts Reports*, 195, 196 (1907). In 1921, Hazel Wedgewood, a former health instructor for the Massachusetts Department of Public Health reported that

this obvious contradiction in the laws has been extremely detrimental to both the midwife and her patient. It has resulted not in eliminating the midwife, but in her practicing more or less surreptitiously, with no help from physicians where it could possibly be avoided, even when such care was imperative for the welfare of the mother and the baby. This contradiction has also resulted in many unregistered births.

Wedgewood, "Midwifery," 73.

33. *Documents*, House of Representatives, Commonwealth of Massachusetts, 1913; *Journal of the House of Representatives*, Commonwealth of Massachusetts, 1913.

34. S. Josephine Baker, "The Function of the Midwife," *Woman's Medical Journal*, 23 (September 1913), 196-197; Levy, "Maternal and Infant," 53; Newmayer, "Status," 718; Marriner, *Midwifery in Alabama*, pp. 1-2, 10; *Report*, Board of Health of Mississippi (1919-1921), p. 198; W. A. Plecker, "The Midwife Problem in Virginia," *Virginia Medical Semi-Monthly*, 19 (December 1914), 457; *First Annual Report*, Massachusetts State Department of Health (1915), p. 25.

35. See, for example, "Section on Midwifery," *Transactions of the American Association for the Study and Prevention of Infant Mortality*,

2 (1911), 163-255; "Section on Midwifery," *Transactions of the American Association for the Study and Prevention of Infant Mortality,* 3 (1912), 219-276.

The AASPIM published the *Transactions* of its annual meetings from its inception in 1910 until its disbandment in 1935. In 1918, the name of the association was changed to the American Child Hygiene Association. In 1923, the American Child Hygiene Association merged with the Child Health Organization of America to form the American Child Health Association.

36. White House Conference on Child Health and Protection, *Obstetric Education* (New York, 1932), p. 169.

5

The Early Twentieth-Century Midwife Debate: Opponents

Most of the opposition to the midwife originated from physicians who felt that the status of obstetrics needed to be upgraded. These physicians, many of whom were obstetric specialists, feared that the obstetrician would never receive due recognition in the "over-crowded" medical profession as long as women, untrained in the medical sciences, continued to serve as birth attendants. Thus, they embarked on a campaign to persuade both the medical profession and the public that obstetrics was a complicated medical specialty requiring the skills of a highly trained physician.

During the second and third decades of the twentieth century, medical journals throughout the United States published a variety of articles on this topic. One of the first, and perhaps most influential, publications of this type appeared in 1911 and was appropriately titled, "The Midwife Problem and Medical Education in the United States." Dr. J. Whitridge Williams, the leading figure in American obstetrics during the early decades of the twentieth century and a professor at the Johns Hopkins University School of Medicine, conducted the study at the request of the newly organized American Association for the Study and Prevention of Infant Mortality. He concluded that medical schools were "inadequately equipped for teaching obstetrics properly." Williams arrived at this conclusion after examining the answers to a lengthy questionnaire that he sent to the professors in 120 medical schools giving a full, four-year course of instruction.[1]

The forty-three professors who responded to the questionnaire appraised the situation with amazing candor. More than one-third of the respondents indicated that they were not obstetric specialists, and several admitted that they could not perform a cesarean section. Only twenty-one of the professors had served in lying-in hospitals before assuming their teaching duties. Twenty-nine of the respondents acknowledged that their hospital equipment was unsatisfactory for teaching obstetrics. Over one-half of the physicians maintained that they had never trained a person whom they felt was competent to become a professor of obstetrics in a first-class medical school. One-fourth of the physicians replied that the "ordinary graduate" was not prepared to practice obstetrics. Perhaps the most startling revelation to come out of the study was that the majority of the professors believed that "general practitioners lose as many and possibly more women from puerperal infection than do midwives."[2]

Because of the "degraded position" of obstetrics in American medical education, Williams hoped that doctors could be "taught to realize that the more difficult [obstetric] operations belong to major surgery, are quite as serious as most operations in abdominal surgery, and often require the greatest skill and experience." So far as the public was concerned, he was adamant that men and women throughout the United States

be taught that a well-conducted hospital is the ideal place for delivery, especially in the case of those with limited incomes. Moreover, they should learn that the average compensation for obstetrical cases is usually quite inadequate . . . and that doctors who are obliged to live from their practice, cannot reasonably be expected to give much better service than they are paid for.[3]

Williams acknowledged that obstetrics would never be designated a complicated medical specialty until a "thorough-going reform" of American medical education was undertaken. He agreed with the *Flexner Report* that there were far too many medical schools in the United States. He estimated that a properly conducted obstetric department of a university-affiliated medical school would need a minimum of $20,000 annually for "the salaries of the professors and necessary assistants and for laboratory expenses, not to mention the cost of maintaining the requisite number of patients."

Such an expensive enterprise could never be offered in "proprietary or pseudo-university medical schools." Williams also pointed out that even reputable medical schools tended to slight the subject of obstetrics. He reported that some of the professors at the Johns Hopkins University School of Medicine, the leading medical institution of the time, were of the opinion that "the obstetrician need only be a man-midwife who is content to eat the crumbs that fall from the rich man's table."[4]

Because Williams regarded obstetrics as a complicated medical specialty, he was "very dubious concerning the possibility of developing satisfactory midwives by any method of instruction." He saw little problem in gradually abolishing midwives in urban areas and replacing them with a "marked extension of lying-in charities." He recognized that it was unrealistic to propose that lying-in hospitals be established in rural areas of the United States where the population was so scattered, but he offered no solution to this dilemma. Williams believed that midwives, if left alone, would eventually be displaced by better trained general practitioners and obstetricians. Until this was accomplished he hoped that other physicians would join him in the campaign to alert the American public to the need for better obstetric care.[5]

Williams's emphasis on the poor state of obstetric education in the United States and the need for it to be developed into a recognized medical specialty was a theme that was often reiterated by midwife opponents between 1910 and 1930. His 1911 study, "The Midwife Problem and Medical Education in the United States," played a prominent role in convincing other physicians to work for the reform of obstetric education and for the abolition of midwives. During the 1910-1920 period this topic was frequently discussed at the annual meetings of the American Association for the Study and Prevention of Infant Mortality. At the 1914 meeting, for instance, George W. Kosmak, a physician at New York Lying-in Hospital, congratulated Williams for alerting the medical profession to the "deplorable condition" of obstetric education. He maintained that most medical faculties regarded obstetrics "as a sort of side issue" because midwives were allowed "to practice an important branch of medicine with a much too brief and unsatisfactory training." Kosmak was also critical of physicians and public health officials who modeled their "ideas on the subject of midwives on those of foreign countries" because the medical profession abroad was "rather dissatisfied with midwives."[6]

At the same meeting, Dr. Joseph B. De Lee, the founder of Chicago Lying-in Hospital (1895) and a leading figure in the movement to eradicate midwives, argued that their legal recognition was proof that "obstetrics is on a low plane." In rhetorical fashion he asked, "Do you wonder that a young man will not adopt this field as his special work? If a delivery requires so little brains and skill that a midwife can conduct it, there is not the place for him." The following year, De Lee presented a paper to the AASPIM in which he expanded this theme. His paper was appropriately titled "Progress Toward Ideal Obstetrics." He urged the medical profession to realize that "parturition, viewed with modern eyes, is no longer a normal function, but that it has imposing pathologic dignity. . . ." He further maintained that only when the science and art of obstetrics were properly appreciated would the midwife "be impossible to mention" and the double standard in obstetrics abandoned.[7]

Charles E. Ziegler, a Pittsburgh obstetrician who was an outspoken opponent of the midwife, reiterated the view that obstetric education could not be reformed "so long as 50 per cent of the cases are in the hands of individuals with a poor preliminary education and as little medical training as have the midwives." In 1912, he told the members of the AASPIM that "we can get along very nicely without the midwife." He was opposed to her training and regulation because he feared that this might enable her to attain a permanent place in the American medical hierarchy. He also accused midwives of monopolizing clinical material and, thereby, compounding the difficulties of those physicians who were interested in elevating the status of obstetrics.[8]

The American Association for the Study and Prevention of Infant Mortality was quite determined in its efforts to alert the medical profession and the public to the potential dangers of childbirth and the need for immediate improvements in obstetric education. When the organization was founded in 1910, a special Section on Midwifery was established. In 1912, its chairwoman, Dr. Mary Sherwood, made it clear that

this is the section on midwifery in its broad sense, not the section on midwives. Its purpose is to determine to what extent present methods of obstetrical practice in America are a factor in preventable infant mortality and what reforms are necessary in order to insure to every infant the right to be well born.

The distinction between midwifery and midwives was made even clearer the following year when the title of the midwifery section was changed to the "Session on Obstetrics."[9]

Between 1911 and 1915, brief reports on the midwife situation in various localities throughout the United States were presented at the annual meetings of the AASPIM. These reports usually included statistical information on the number of practicing midwives as well as assessments of their work. For example, reports issued for Maine for the years 1911-1913 indicated that the midwife rarely served as the attendant at birth. In 1913, Dr. H. J. Everett of Portland, Maine, reported that .5 percent of all births in the state were attended by midwives.[10]

The vast majority of the papers presented to the AASPIM, as well as the debates and discussions that ensued, dealt with ways to improve the quality of obstetric education. From time to time midwife proponents made themselves heard. Dr. S. Josephine Baker, a staunch supporter of the midwife, was present at many of the annual meetings of the association. In 1911, she delivered a paper, "Schools for Midwives," in which she endorsed the concept of the trained and regulated midwife. She also defended the midwife on those occasions when roundtable discussions on obstetrics were held.[11] As time progressed, however, the association devoted less and less attention to the midwife. In 1918, its name was changed to the American Child Hygiene Association and its scope was expanded to include sessions on child welfare, pediatrics, education, juvenile delinquency, and adolescent problems.[12]

During the 1910-1920 period, the American Association for the Study and Prevention of Infant Mortality published numerous papers on the need to elevate the status of obstetrics. Although its membership was relatively small, the results of many of its studies and investigations were circulated to a large segment of the medical profession.[13] Several of the papers that were originally published in the *Transactions* later appeared in medical journals with a wider circulation, such as the *American Journal of Obstetrics and the Diseases of Women and Children* and the *Journal of the American*

Medical Association.[14] The republication of these papers most certainly influenced other physicians to write similar articles.

Medical practitioners were still making references to J. Whitridge Williams's paper on the poor level of obstetric education in the United States four years after it was first published. Dr. John F. Moran, in an article published in the *Journal of the American Medical Association* in 1915, bemoaned the fact that few of the recommendations suggested by Williams had been implemented. Moran, who served as president of the Washington Obstetrical and Gynecological Society, repeated the very familiar argument that "obstetrics is the most arduous, least appreciated, least supported, and least compensated of all the branches of medicine." He was adamant that motherhood be "zealously guarded and cared for by trained physicians and not by ignorant midwives. . . ." He also urged the medical profession to awaken the public to the "clinical fact that normal pregnancy and parturition are the exception. . . ."[15] Similar arguments were expressed in various regional medical journals. Writing for the *Illinois Medical Journal* in 1920, Dr. Rudolph W. Holmes demanded, "How can the crude mind of a midwife appreciate the gravity of an impending eclampsia, a contracted pelvis, or heart disease, etc., and secure adequate assistants at any early moment?"[16]

The introduction of Twilight Sleep into the United States around 1914 tended to support the view that obstetrics was a complicated medical specialty. Twilight Sleep was a new method of "painless childbirth," perfected by physicians in Freiburg, Germany, a few years before World War I. It consisted of a light sleep, induced by an injection of morphine and the amnesiac drug, scopolamine, upon the onset of labor. When it was properly administered, the pregnant woman delivered her baby with no memory of pain.[17]

At first, American physicians were reluctant to provide women with Twilight Sleep because they were unsure of its safety. Many prospective mothers, however, were quite adamant that they be able to experience "painless childbirth." Dr. Elizabeth Taylor Ransom, a Boston physician, helped popularize this new method by establishing the first Twilight Sleep Maternity Hospital in the United States in 1914. Shortly thereafter, other American doctors adopted the technique.[18] Physicians who were concerned about elevating the status of obstetrics, such as Joseph B. De Lee, did not hesitate to point out that Twilight Sleep should only be "practiced by special-istically trained obstetricians in specially equipped maternity hospi-tals, with an abundance of trained assistants and nurses. . . ." De Lee was also grateful that popular magazines were publishing arti-cles on Twilight Sleep, for they were drawing "the attention of the public to child-bearing women and their sufferings and necessities." Similarly, Dr. Mary Sherwood was optimistic that the publicity surrounding Twilight Sleep would encourage the laity to demand better obstetric care.[19]

Another obstetric innovation that supported the view that child-birth was a potentially dangerous phenomenon, requiring the services of the skilled physician, was the "prophylactic forceps operation." Joseph B. De Lee, who presented a paper on this topic to the 1920 annual meeting of the American Gynecological Society, was the first physician to suggest the operation. De Lee defined the prophylactic forceps operation as "the routine delivery of the child in head presentation, where the head has come to rest on the pelvic floor. . . ." He recommended that "primiparous labors and those in which the condition of the soft parts approximates a first labor" be delivered in this manner in combination with Twilight Sleep. He defended it on the grounds that it lessened the pain and suffering of the parturient woman, preserved the "integrity of the pelvic floor," and saved "babies' brains from injuries." De Lee admitted that, perhaps, there were already too many forceps operations being performed by unskilled general practitioners, but he felt that "in skillful hands the danger [from the operation] is nil." He wanted to "bring the general practice of obstetrics up to the level of the special-ist . . . not bring the ideals of obstetrics down to the level of general, the occasional practitioner."[20]

The incidence of cesarean sections also increased dramatically during the first three decades of the twentieth century. At the be-ginning of this period, abdominal delivery was practiced only on those rare occasions when specific complications, such as a con-tracted pelvis or obstructed birth canal, occurred. By 1930, the cesarean section was being performed for "every imaginable com-plication of pregnancy and labor," including the "desire of the patient."[21] One enthusiastic physician reported an incidence of one cesarean for every fourteen births he attended, while conservative obstetricians reported rates from one in forty to one in eighty.[22]

The 1930 White House Conference on Child Health and Protection conducted a survey of 119 American hospitals which revealed that 2.9 percent of all deliveries were performed by cesarean section. This was substantially higher than that reported by many of the leading European maternity hospitals. At the Stockholm Lying-in Hospital, as an example, abdominal deliveries made up a mere .06 percent of the total number of deliveries. By the close of this period, the cesarean section had become fashionable, and many physicians confidently accepted the dictum, "once a cesarean, always a cesarean." Like the prophylactic forceps operations, only a highly trained physician was capable of safely and successfully performing the cesarean section.[23]

As artificial delivery became increasingly frequent, the number of hospital-delivered births grew as well. Many physicians were hopeful that all deliveries would eventually occur in hospitals. J. Whitridge Williams had argued that the "well-conducted hospital is the ideal place for delivery, especially in the case of those with limited incomes." Other physicians concurred in this opinion. In 1914, Dr. Edward P. Davis presented a paper to the American Association for the Study and Prevention of Infant Mortality in which he expressed concern over the fact that "in obstetrics less use is made of hospitals than in other branches of medicine, and with great loss to the community and increase in suffering and mortality." He believed that women should always be hospitalized for first confinements because "surgical aid is required in a much larger percentage of cases than in subsequent confinements, and perfect recovery is only possible with good surgical care."[24]

Although many early twentieth-century physicians argued that the hospital was the ideal place for delivery, most women chose to have their babies at home. Many poor women avoided the charity hospitals, because they feared they would be subjected to experimentation and obstetric interference. Women of moderate means could not afford the high costs of hospitalization. Only the wealthy woman, who could afford the price of a private room and the fee of the obstetrician, willingly entered the hospital.[25]

In addition, there was a simple logistical reason why so few births occurred in hospitals during the early years of the twentieth century. Prior to 1910, there were not enough hospitals in existence to take care of large numbers of maternity cases. The rapid rate of growth of American hospitals did not get underway until the second decade of the twentieth century. For example, the bed capacity of American hospitals increased from 421,065 in 1909 to 755,722 in 1923. By 1933, this figure had increased to 1,027,046.[26]

Before the advent of the automobile, it was also extremely difficult to get the parturient woman to the hospital in time for its obstetric services to be of any use to her. In an article published in the *Southern Medical Journal* in 1939, Dr. J. McF. Bergland related an account of the problems he had experienced thirty-five years earlier when it became necessary to move an obstetric patient from her home to the nearby Johns Hopkins Hospital. Since it took almost one hour to get the ambulance out, the senior attending physician suggested that the 160-pound patient be manually carried by two male attendants the short distance to the hospital.[27]

The number of hospital-delivered births increased rapidly after 1910. Although few reliable statistics exist for the early years of the twentieth century, a 1916 survey conducted by the New York City Department of Health indicated that 19.1 percent of all births in the borough of Manhattan occurred in hospitals. Presumably, this rate was much higher than that occurring in less populated cities and towns. The Children's Bureau reported in 1921 that hospital confinements occurred much more frequently in cities than in rural areas. In Baltimore, for example, 18.7 percent of all births took place in hospitals "as compared with only 2.6 percent of the births in Maryland outside of Baltimore." In 1935, the year that the first national statistics on hospital deliveries were published, 36.9 percent of all births were reported to have taken place in hospitals.[28]

The campaign in behalf of hospital delivery gathered momentum during the 1930s. For example, in 1934 the New York Obstetrical Society issued a statement in opposition to home delivery. It maintained "that delivery in a well-organized and well-equipped hospital is safer than home delivery." The society argued that obstetrics was no longer "a one man job" and that, consequently, "home deliveries should not be encouraged, unless they can be conducted with every safeguard of medical supervision, equipment and assistance." By 1940, over one-half of all births were attended by physicians in hospitals.[29]

The efforts of physicians to elevate the status of obstetrics to that of a recognized medical specialty were partially realized in 1930 with the establishment of the American Board of Obstetrics and Gynecology. According to the Articles of Incorporation, the board was formed in order "to grant and to insure to physicians, duly licensed by law, certificates or other equivalent recognition of special knowledge of obstetrics and gynecology." The first certification exams were given in 1931. Sixty-five of the original seventy-nine applicants were successful in qualifying for recognition as specialists. Both medical historians and physicians agree that the establishment of the board "exerted a powerful influence" in the elevation of obstetrics and gynecology as a specialty.[30]

The need to raise the status of obstetrics was the theme most often reiterated by those physicians who wanted to bring about the demise of the midwife. Many of the other anti-midwife arguments they originated also related to the degrated position of the obstetrician. For example, a frequent complaint expressed by physicians was that they were poorly reimbursed for their obstetric services. Many doctors feared that this trend would continue as long as midwives persisted in attending 50 percent of all the births for less than one-half the fee charged by medical practitioners.[31] It was quite natural for them to call for the elimination of the midwife on the grounds that she posed an economic threat to the medical profession. Abolishing the midwife appeared to be a partial solution to the problem of "overcrowding." Moreover, the clinical material that she monopolized was "necessary for the proper training of medical students." James L. Huntington, a prominent anti-midwife critic who was a physician at Boston Lying-in Hospital, chastised the midwife for contributing "nothing to the knowledge of obstetrics" and losing the "details of half of the obstetrical cases." Until adequate clinical material was available, many physicians believed there was little chance for obstetrics to receive its due recognition.[32]

Most physicians who favored the elimination of the midwife agreed with J. Whitridge Williams that she should be replaced by a "marked extension of lying-in charities." Charels E. Ziegler was one of several physicians who elaborated on this idea. In his paper, "The Elimination of the Midwife," Ziegler stated that obstetric charities should consist of both maternity hospitals and maternity dispensaries, which were "a part of, or closely affiliated with, a medical school." The hospital would provide care for all those who could not "secure proper attention at home," while the dispensary would aid women who were delivered in their own domiciles. Ziegler estimated that the births attended by New York City midwives in 1912 could be handled through "maternity dispensaries for an additional expenditure of not over $100,000, provided such dispensaries received as much in fees as the midwives now do." James L. Huntington figured that obstetric charities could actually pay for themselves. He reported that the outpatients of Boston Lying-in Hospital paid an average of $1.28 per delivery in 1910. This fee covered all the expenses of the Outpatient Department and left it with a budget surplus of $807.82. In 1911, the average fee of $1.27 per delivery produced a surplus of $833.31.[33]

J. Clifton Edgar, a physician from New York City, also favored the replacement of midwives by obstetric charities. He emphasized that this

need not cause any great hardship, for most of the better class of midwives now in existence could subsequently find a livelihood, . . . in caring for the older children and the household during the mother's two weeks absence in a maternity hospital, or during the time the mother is confined to her bed in her own home under the care of a dispensary physician.[34]

The replacement of midwives by maternity dispensaries and hospitals was especially welcomed by physicians who were concerned about providing medical students with adequate clinical material. Charles E. Ziegler estimated that the marked extension of hospitals and dispensaries would enable every student to attend at least fifty births before going into private practice. Other physicians were also hopeful that the establishment of additional maternity hospitals would substantially improve the clinical training of medical students.[35]

Not everyone was satisfied with the clinical experiences provided by maternity dispensaries. As early as 1918, Dr. Edward P. Davis, a professor at the Jefferson Medical College in Philadelphia, characterized the "so-called out-patient practice in obstetrics in hospitals and dispensaries" as a "relic of bygone days." He argued that the obstetric student should no more be sent out into the "filthy" tenements than the students of surgery. He felt that prospective obstetricians should be trained in hospital wards, "under the most favorable conditions and best possible appliances." Only when enough hospitals were established to accommodate the population and students would infant mortality "be considerably lessened and medical education greatly improved." Davis did not totally rule out the possibility of home delivery, but he favored it only when physicians were "able and willing to install hospital facilities in private houses, [and] to employ a sufficient number of assistants and nurses to maintain hospital techniques. . . ."[36]

The problem of finding a substitute for the rural midwife was much more complicated. Many southern physicians reluctantly conceded that she was a "necessary evil" because "the distances are too great" and "the fees are too small to support a greater number of physicians." A 1928 study of the midwife situation in Virginia, conducted by Dr. Greer Baughman, professor of obstetrics at Virginia Medical College, concluded that "the doctors would work themselves to death and die broke" if they attempted to deliver all the rural births. Southern physicians were further dismayed because "in the South we have to deal with the ignorant and superstitious negro [sic]," while in the Northeast midwives "are either foreign or of foreign parentage and a fair percentage of them have been trained in Europe or at the school [Bellevue] in New York."[37]

In a paper delivered to the 1924 annual meeting of the Southern Medical Association, Dr. C. R. Hardin of Lumberton, North Carolina, summarized the sentiments of the anti-midwife physicians of the South in the following manner: "Since the evil cannot be eradicated, the danger to the public can be minimized by some provision for the proper regulation, supervision, and control of the midwife by the state." If these provisions were properly carried out, Hardin was hopeful that they would lead to her ultimate elimination. Until her demise, the midwife would continue to exert a negative "moral effect upon obstetric standards."[38]

Anti-midwife physicians were well aware of the high infant and maternal mortality rates in the United States. Although they spared no words in describing the "ignorant" and "dirty" ways of the midwife, they did not hold her totally responsible for this excessive number of deaths. Arthur B. Emmons and James L. Huntington, two Boston physicians who co-authored several articles on the midwife, described her as "ignorant of the situation . . . unprincipled, anxious only for the fee, and callous of the feelings and welfare of her patients. She looks upon her work as a legitimate form of livelihood, not as an enabling profession." Nevertheless, Emmons and Huntington believed that American obstetricians were ultimately responsible for this poor state of affairs because they "are the final authority to set the standard and lead the way to safety. They alone can properly educate the medical profession, the legislators, and the public."[39]

Many physicians admitted that the general practitioner often did as much harm as the midwife. J. Whitridge Williams's 1911 study revealed that medical professors throughout the United States were in agreement on this point. Some physicians criticized the family doctor for "cling[ing] to even the difficult cases in obstetrics with a jealous tenacity"; others went so far as to make no distinction between the practices of the "unworthy" general practitioner and the midwife. Dr. Edward P. Davis maintained that they both attempt "to prevent the loss of personal gain" by prejudicing "ignorant persons" against hospital deliveries and surgical operations. Another physician wrote of the "dirty and untrained" midwife and her "accomplice, the doctor, usually ignorant and often unscrupulous."[40]

The fact that the general practitioner had as poor, or even poorer, a record than the midwife was just one more reason why many physicians favored her elimination. Charles E. Ziegler readily admitted that "large numbers of physicians do equally as poor obstetrics as the midwives." He believed that the sensible way to solve this dilemma was to "train the physician until he is capable of doing good obstetrics and then make it financially possible for him to do it, by eliminating the midwife."[41] Similarly, Dr. George W. Kosmak argued that "there is no valid reason to accede to the demand for the midwife as an institution . . . [because] there are doctors who do not do as well, or who do worse, than this personage." Kosmak, like most other anti-midwife physicians, was of the opinion that obstetrics belonged "to the scientifically trained physician and to none else." If obstetric work were poorly performed, it should be corrected; under no circumstances should a program be developed that might lead to the institutionalization of the midwife.[42]

Physicians were especially disturbed at the thought of the midwife attaining a permanent place within the American medical hierarchy. She was perceived as an "outside influence" who wanted to invade the "legitimate field of medicine." It was quite common for anti-midwife physicians to compare her with other "irregular" practitioners, such as osteopaths, optometrists, and Christian Scientists.[43] Most importantly, specialists, such as J. Whitridge Williams, were optimistic that general practitioners could be taught to refer complicated cases to properly equipped lying-in hospitals. By establishing such a referral system within the established medical profession, the threat of any "outside influence" would be abolished and obstetricians would have additional clinical material with which to train their professional successors better.[44]

Many of the criticisms heaped upon the midwife resulted from the anti-immigrant and anti-Negro prejudices of the period. William R. Nicholson, a Philadelphia physician, argued in 1917 that the midwife problem in the United States was due to the "unrestricted immigration of the past years, with the consequent establishment of colonies in every large city, as well as in many rural communities." He characterized these newly arrived immigrants as "ignorant in every sense of the word, who do not speak English, who have but little money, but are prolific breeders, and who come here with definite and fixed ideas in favor of the midwife rather than the doctor." Likewise, Dr. George W. Goler, health officer of Rochester, New York, insisted that "the whole midwife problem in America is an attempt to engraft an old continental custom upon the people of the United States." Many physicians were quite pessimistic about the possibility of training immigrants "to resort to maternities and to give up the midwife." Dr. J. M. Baldy pointed out that one hardly makes "a beginning in this educational feature, before there is a new influx and again a new one, ad infinitum." He felt that the one effective way of accomplishing this end was "to stop immigration and we all know how helpless is that task."[45]

Joseph B. De Lee's opposition to the midwife was also colored by racial prejudice. He disapproved of training programs for midwives because they merely provided "a little better care for the poor, the ignorant woman or foreigner." He felt it was impracticable to devote time and energy to a program that only improved the obstetric care of that 40 percent of the population that employed midwives. He wanted to see more emphasis placed on bettering the education of the physicians who attended the births of middle-class and well-to-do Americans.[46]

Racial prejudice predictably played a prominent role in the anti-midwife arguments developed by southern physicians. Dr. Felix J. Underwood, who served as the director of the Bureau of Child Hygiene for Mississippi during the early 1920s, described the conditions surrounding the birth of black infants in the South as follows:

What could be a more pitiable picture than that of a prospective mother housed in an unsanitary home and attended in this most critical period by an accoucheur, filthy and ignorant, and not far removed from the jungles of Africa, laden with its atmosphere of weird superstition and voodooism?[47]

Dr. O. R. Thompson of Macon, Georgia, wrote that southern midwives were much more difficult to train than their northern counterparts because they were primarily "ignorant" and "superstitious" Negroes. In similar fashion, Dr. W. A. Plecker, registrar of the Office of Vital Statistics in Virginia, maintained that the "presumption of these ignorant creatures is simply appalling."[48]

In discussing their reasons for opposing midwives, the opponents did not find it necessary to employ the often-repeated allegation that women were biologically and intellectually inferior to men. By the early twentieth century, the distinctions between the functions of the midwife and the physician were clearly delineated. The education and training that was required of the midwife, even if she attended the Bellevue School for Midwives, was much less rigorous than that required of the physician. Thus, a woman did not have to be a man's equal in order to become a midwife. The question at issue was *not* whether women were qualified to be midwives, but whether anyone, other than a highly trained medical practitioner, was capable of practicing obstetrics competently. The question of whether early twentieth-century male physicians believed women had the ability to become competent medical practitioners is, of course, a separate subject.[49]

Opponents of the midwife disagreed as to whether she should be immediately or gradually eliminated. Anti-midwife physicians in Boston were quite adamant that she be promptly discarded. A 1915 nationwide survey, conducted to determine the reaction of various people to the "midwife problem," revealed that Boston represented the "stronghold of . . . the anti-midwife attitude."[50] Two of the most ouspoken critics of the midwife, Arthur B. Emmons and James L. Huntington, were from Boston. These two physicians wrote numerous articles in which they called for the immediate end of the midwife.[51] In 1913, Huntington also worked with the New England Sub-Committee on Obstetrics of the American Association for the Study and Prevention of Infant Mortality in its successful campaign to prevent the passage of a bill before the Massachusetts legislature which would have provided for the registration of midwives.[52] Since Massachusetts was the only state that outlawed midwives, it was quite natural for its capital city to become the "stronghold of . . . the anti-midwife attitude." The existence of numerous hospitals, medical schools, and research facilities in the Boston area also served to advance the position that obstetrics was a complicated medical specialty for which the midwife was unsuited.[53]

Other critics of the midwife felt that it was impractical to call for her *immediate* elimination. They concluded that she would be a "necessary evil" for many years to come. The leading northern spokesman for this viewpoint was J. Clifton Edgar, a New York City physician. In one of his earliest articles on this topic, Edgar wrote that "since the evil [i.e., the midwife] cannot be eradicated, the dangers to the public must be minimized by some provision for the proper regulation, supervision, and control of the midwife by the state and for her training to do her work in a cleanly and intelligent manner. . . ."[54] Edgar cited the success of the Bellevue School for Midwives as proof that "ignorant" women could be competently trained. Nevertheless, he considered the education of midwives to be a *temporary* measure which should be discontinued as soon as an adequate number of properly trained physicians and obstetricians were produced. In the same article in which Edgar praised the work of the Bellevue School, he also called for "the ultimate elimination of the midwife."[55]

Dr. S. W. Newmayer, head of the Division of Child Hygiene in Philadelphia, was in basic agreement with Edgar. In 1909, Newmayer was assigned the duty of examining and licensing every midwife in Philadelphia. He adopted a very liberal policy and granted as many licenses as possible because he felt it was more important to keep "strict supervision over the midwives" than to refuse them licenses and run the risk of "their practicing without such license or supervision." Although Newmayer worked long and hard to develop a training and regulatory program for Philadelphia midwives, he was basically opposed to their existence. He argued that the "midwife today in the United States is a useless institution." He reluctantly favored the enactment of laws which would protect the public "against the incompetent and daring midwife" because he felt it was presently impossible to train the "foreign mother" to the advantages of obtaining proper obstetric care.[56]

Many southern opponents of the midwife also considered it impractical to demand her immediate elimination. They recognized that it would be many years before it would be possible to replace the southern "granny" with properly qualified physicians and maternity hospitals and dispensaries.[57] Realizing that large segments of the population would receive no obstetric care if the midwife were abolished, many southern state boards of health began cautious experiments for her training and regulation during the 1920s. For the most part, these programs were perceived as stopgap measures. For example, Alabama began investigating the activities of its midwives in 1918. By 1925, a policy of midwifery regulation had developed which was centered in the county health departments. Despite this relatively successful regulatory program, the director of the Alabama Child Hygiene and Public Health Nursing Division was of the opinion that "it is possible to eliminate midwife practice entirely."[58] Similarly, the director of the Mississippi Bureau of Child Welfare stated in 1920 that "the plan is to gradually raise the standard [of the midwife] with the idea of ultimate elimination, when hospital facilities and trained physicians are available in every community." Meanwhile, public health nurses were appointed to travel to the various Mississippi counties in order to conduct midwifery classes and investigate the qualificatons of the candidates.[59]

Like many other southern health officials, Dr. W. A. Plecker, registrar of the Office of Vital Statistics in Virginia, believed the midwife would "remain a necessary evil, with but little hope of general improvement in her methods . . . for a long time." Despite this rather gloomy prognosis, Plecker played an instrumental role in developing a program for the training and regulation of Virginia midwives. He worked diligently to convince physicians to cooperate with the Virginia health department in securing accurate birth and death statistics. He also urged doctors to come to the aid of pregnant "women in distress, regardless of financial reward."[60]

Many of the anti-midwife arguments developed by physicians eventually made their way into the popular magazines of the period. The *Delineator, Good Housekeeping, Ladies' Home Journal,* and *McClure's* were just a few of the magazines that published articles on the high infant and maternal mortality rates in the United States.[61] Both the poorly trained medical practitioner and the midwife were blamed for this predicament. The message implicit in most of these articles was that the obstetric specialist made the best birth attendant. Woods Hutchinson argued in a 1914 article published in *Good Housekeeping* that "if one is content with an eighty percent or four-to-one probability of a successful issue, then the midwife will serve. But if one wants to reach the lowest possible percentage of risk—so low as almost to approach absolute safety—the expert must be utilized." Similarly, *McClure's* published an article in 1915 which compared "the danger from the practice of obstetrics by unskilled general practitioners . . . with that from the practice of midwifery."[62]

A variety of articles appeared which stressed the relationship between proper prenatal care and the reduction of maternal and infant deaths. Special "tips" for pregnant women were usually included in publications of this type. One such article, published in the October 1926 issue of the *Delineator,* was written by the outspoken midwife oponent Joseph B. De Lee. Not surprisingly, he was critical of the practices of midwives, and he advised women to employ competent physicians during pregnancy and parturition.[63] Studies of Twilight Sleep were also published in some of these same women's magazines of the period. The authors of these studies adamantly insisted that only highly trained physicians were capable of administering this new method of "painless childbirth."[64]

Popular magazines also carried feature stories which often chastised the midwife for being "ignorant," "dirty," and "superstitious." One article accused her of causing numerous maternal and infant deaths. On another occasion, the "superstitions" of southern "grannies" were discussed. Nevertheless, the authors generally agreed that comprehensive training programs were capable of substantially improving the midwife's status.[65] Because of the negative view of the midwife presented in these articles, one must question whether or not they motivated the public to support training and regulation. They may very well have served to reinforce the popular prejudices held against the midwife.

The campaign against the midwife was widespread and well publicized. Opponents spared no words in denouncing her "dirty" and "ignorant" ways. They delivered papers on this topic to the annual meetings of the various medical societies established throughout the United States. These papers, as well as other articles, were often published in the major medical journals of the period. The American Association for the Study and Prevention of Infant Mortality devoted a great deal of its time and energy to elevating the status of obstetrics and vilifying the midwife. Many of the state and municipal bureaus of child hygiene also felt that she should be ultimately eliminated. Finally, popular magazines published articles that contained acrid criticisms of the midwife.

The height of the anti-midwife campaign occurred between 1910 and 1920. By the 1920s, much of the original furor had tapered off. Members of the American Child Hygiene Association (the successor to the AASPIM) rarely discussed the issue of the midwife. The agenda of the annual meetings of the association included a variety of child-related topics, such as juvenile delinquency, education, and adolescent problems. Medical journals and popular periodicals also published fewer articles on the "midwife problem" after 1920. The major reason for this change of focus was that fewer and fewer births were being attended by midwives. Reports from throughout the United States indicated that the ranks of the midwives were sharply and steadily decreasing. In 1909, midwives in New York City attended 40.55 percent of all births. By 1920, this figure had dropped to 26.6 percent. There were 712 practicing midwives in New Jersey in 1918. Nine years later, this number had been reduced to 399. Midwives in Birmingham, Alabama, attended 968 births in 1917;

in 1924 they attended only 10 babies.[66] The same story is true for other areas.

The critics of the midwife were partially responsible for the reduction of her numbers. There were a variety of other factors that also contributed to her demise. An examination of the tactics and arguments of the midwife proponents will reveal what many of these were.

NOTES

1. J. Whitridge Williams, "The Midwife Problem and Medical Education in the United States," *Transactions of the American Association for the Study and Prevention of Infant Mortality,* 2 (1911), 166. A condensed version of this article was published under the title "Medical Education and the Midwife Problem in the United States," *Journal of the American Medical Association,* 58 (January 1912), 1-7.

2. Williams, "The Midwife Problem," 165, 167, 174, 175, 176, 178, 179.

3. Ibid., 188, 189, 190.

Similar lamentations about speciality status and training were found in medical areas other than obstetrics during the late nineteenth and early twentieth centuries. The development of specialist societies and organizations and the response of general practitioners to medical specialization are detailed in Rosemary Stevens, *American Medicine and the Public Interest* (New Haven, Conn., 1971), pp. 34-97.

4. Williams, "The Midwife Problem," 184, 185, 186, 187, 188.

5. Ibid., 192-193.

6. "Discussion—George W. Kosmak," *Transactions of the American Association for the Study and Prevention of Infant Mortality,* 5 (1914), 203. Arthur B. Emmóns and James L. Huntington devoted a great deal of attention to the disadvantages of the European midwife system. See, for example, Emmons and Huntington, "Has the Trained and Supervised Midwife Made Good?" *Transactions of the American Association for the Study and Prevention of Infant Mortality,* 2 (1911), 199-206; Emmons and Huntington, "Review of the Midwife Situation," *Boston Medical and Surgical Journal,* 164 (1911), 251-255.

7. Joseph B. De Lee, "Report of Sub-Committee for Illinois," *Transactions of the American Association for the Study and Prevention of Infant Mortality,* 5 (1914), 231; Joseph B. De Lee, "Progress Toward Ideal Obstetrics," *Transactions of the American Association for the Study and Prevention of Infant Mortality,* 6 (1915), 117; "Childbirth: Nature vs. Drugs," *Time,* 2 (May 1936), 38.

8. Charles E. Ziegler, "The Elimination of the Midwife," *Transactions of the American Association for the Study and Prevention of Infant Mortality*, 3 (1912), 222-223, 258. A condensed version of this article was published in the *Journal of the American Medical Association*, 60 (January 1913), 32-38.

9. Mary Sherwood, "Statement by the Chairman, Section on Midwifery," *Transactions of the American Association for the Study and Prevention of Infant Mortality*, 3 (1912), 218; "Session on Obstetrics," *Transactions of the American Association for the Study and Prevention of Infant Mortality*, 4 (1913), 173.

10. "Midwives in New England," *Transactions of the American Association for the Study and Prevention of Infant Mortality*, 4 (1913), 233. Since midwives attended approximately 50 percent of the births in the United States at the turn of the twentieth century, it is quite likely that Everett underestimated the percentage of midwife-attended births in Maine. The state department of health did not conduct any special midwife investigations during the early years of the twentieth century. Thus, Everett was apparently forced to rely on his own research. The rural makeup of the Maine population may have caused him to overlook those women who occasionally aided a parturient friend or relative, but who did not consider themselves to be midwives. *Bulletins*, Maine State Department of Health (1905-1922).

11. S. Josephine Baker, "Schools for Midwives," *Transactions of the American Association for the Study and Prevention of Infant Mortality*, 2 (1911), 241; "Discussion," *Transactions of the American Association for the Study and Prevention of Infant Mortality*, 2 (1912), 253-255.

12. "Report," *Transactions of the American Child Hygiene Association*, 9 (1918), 14.

13. In 1911, the total membership of the AASPIM was 525. By 1916, the ranks of the association had more than doubled to 1,110 members. The 1920 membership totaled 1,232. "Report," *Transactions of the American Association for the Study and Prevention of Infant Mortality*, 2 (1911), 15; "Report," *Transactions of the American Association for the Study and Prevention of Infant Mortality*, 7 (1916), 14; "Report," *Transactions of the American Child Hygiene Association*, 11 (1920), 13.

14. For example, see notes 1, 8, this chapter; Baker, "Schools for Midwives" was also published in the *American Journal of Obstetrics and the Diseases of Women and Children*, 65 (1912), 256-270; a condensed version of Arthur B. Emmons and James L. Huntington, "Has the Trained and Supervised Midwife Made Good?" was published in the *American Journal of Obstetrics and the Diseases of Women and Children*, 65 (March 1912), 393-404 under the title, "The Midwife: Her Future in the United States";

J. Clifton Edgar, "The Education, Licensing and Supervision of the Midwife," *Transactions of the American Association for the Study and Prevention of Infant Mortality*, 6 (1915), 90-104, was also published in the *American Journal of Obstetrics and the Diseases of Women and Children*, 73 (March 1916), 385-398; J. M. Baldy, "Is the Midwife a Necessity?" *Transactions of the American Association for the Study and Prevention of Infant Mortality*, (1915), 105-113, was also published in the *American Journal of Obstetrics and the Diseases of Women and Children*, 73 (March 1916), 399-407.

15. John F. Moran, "The Endowment of Motherhood," *Journal of the American Medical Association*, 64 (January 1915), 125-126.

16. Rudolph W. Holmes, "Midwife Practice: An Anachronism," *Illinois Medical Journal*, 37 (January 1920), 29. See also Edwin Gragin, "The Present Status of Modern Obstetrics," *Journal of the Maine Medical Association*, 3 (February 1913), 1175; Elizabeth Shaver, "Infant Mortality and the Midwife Problem," *Louisville (Kentucky) Monthly Journal of Medicine and Surgery*, 19 (June 1912), 26; Walter E. Welz, "Michigan's Midwife Problem," *Journal of the Michigan State Medical Society*, 21 (December 1912), 792; James L. Huntington, "The Midwife in Massachusetts: Her Anomalous Position," *Boston Medical and Surgical Journal*, 168 (March 1913), 419.

17. Marguerite Tracy and Constance Leupp, "Painless Childbirth," *McClure's*, 43 (June 1914), 37-39.

18. "Is the Twilight Sleep Safe—For Me?" *Woman's Home Companion*, 42 (January 1915), 10, 43; Constance Leupp and Burton J. Hendrick, "Twilight Sleep in America," *McClure's*, 44 (April 1915), 25-26; Richard Wertz and Dorothy Wertz, "Lying-in, A History of Childbirth in America: Its Technologies and Social Relations," (Boston, unpublished manuscript, [1974]), [41-43].

19. Leupp and Hendrick, "Twilight Sleep," 37; De Lee, "Report of Sub-Committee for Illinois," 231; "Discussion," *Transactions of the American Association for the Study and Prevention of Infant Mortality*, 6 (1915), 158.

20. Joseph B. De Lee, "The Prophylactic Forceps Operation," *American Journal of Obstetrics and Gynecology*, 1 (1920), 34, 43-44.

21. White House Conference on Child Health and Protection, *Fetal, Newborn, and Maternal Morbidity and Mortality* (New York, 1933), p. 231.

22. Ward F. Seeley, "Effects of Interference in Obstetrical Cases," *American Journal of Public Health*, 15 (January 1925), 24.

23. White House Conference, *Fetal*, pp. 231-236; Stevens, *American Medicine*, pp. 200-201.

24. Williams, "The Midwife Problem," 190; Edward P. Davis, "The Need

of Hospitals for Maternity Surgical Cases," *Transactions of the American Association for the Study and Prevention of Infant Mortality*, 5 (1914), 196-197. See also Huntington, "The Midwife in Massachusetts," 421; Edgar, "The Education," 95; Josiah Morris Slemons, *The Prospective Mother: A Handbook for Women During Pregnancy* (New York, 1912), pp. 232-235.

25. George W. Kosmak, "Maternity Hospital Care for the Woman of Moderate Means," *Transactions of the American Association for the Study and Prevention of Infant Mortality*, 4 (1913), 208; Davis, "The Need of Hospitals," 196-201.

26. E. H. L. Corwin, *The American Hospital* (New York, 1946), p. 8.

27. J. McF. Bergland, "Changes in Obstetrical Procedure During the Last Thirty-five Years," *Southern Medical Journal*, 32 (1939), 188.

28. Lee W. Thomas, "The Supervision of Midwives in New York City," *Monthly Bulletin*, Department of Health, City of New York, 9 (May 1919), 117; Robert M. Woodbury, *Maternal Mortality: The Risk of Death in Childbirth and From All Diseases Caused by Pregnancy and Confinement*, United States Department of Labor, Children's Bureau Publication, No. 158 (Washington, D.C., 1926), p. 54; Elizabeth Tandy, *Infant and Maternal Mortality Among Negroes*, United States Department of Labor, Children's Bureau Publication, No. 243 (Washington, D.C., 1937), p. 7.

29. Hazel Corbin, "Historical Development of Nurse-Midwifery in this Country, and Present Trends," *Bulletin of the American College of Nurse-Midwifery*, 4 (March 1959), 15; *Report of the Committee of the New York Obstetrical Society to Review the Maternal Mortality Report of the Public Health Relations Committee of the New York Academy of Medicine* (New York, 1934), p. 7; United States Bureau of the Census, *Statistical Abstract of the United States: 1973* (Washington, D.C., 1973), p. 52.

30. Walter Dannreuther, "The American Board of Obstetrics and Gynecology: Its Origin, Progress, and Accomplishments," *American Journal of Obstetrics and Gynecology*, 68 (July 1954), 16-17, 19; Robert F. Monroe, "Historical Development of Obstetric Education in the South," *Southern Medical Journal*, 52 (1959), 1144; Craig W. Muckle, "The First Five Years: A History of the Beginnings of the American Academy of Obstetrics and Gynecology," *Obstetrics and Gynecology*, 13 (March 1959), 365.

The work of the American Board of Obstetrics and Gynecology must be distinguished from that of the American Gynecological Society (1876) and the American Association of Obstetricians and Gynecologists (1888). These latter two organizations were, for the most part, scientific societies devoted to scholarly research in the area of obstetrics and gynecology. Unlike the American Board of Obstetrics and Gynecology, they were not regulatory agencies. Stevens, *American Medicine*, p. 54; Houston S. Everett, "The History of the American Gynecological Society Prepared for the Celebration of the 100th Anniversary of Its Founding in 1876" (unpublished paper, 1974).

31. Moran, "Endowment," 125; A. K. Paine, "The Midwife Problem," *Boston Medical and Surgical Journal*, 173 (November 1915), 761; Williams, "The Midwife Problem," 190; Ziegler, "The Elimination of the Midwife," 222-234, 226.

Statistics comparing the fees of physicians and midwives may be found in Louis S. Reed, *Midwives, Chiropodists, and Optometrists: Their Place in Medical Care* (Chicago, 1932), p. 17.

32. Ziegler, "The Elimination of the Midwife," 226; Huntington, "The Midwife in Massachusetts," 420.

33. Ziegler, "The Elimination of the Midwife," 231, 235; Huntington, "The Midwife in Massachusetts," 421.

34. Edgar, "The Education," 95. Other physicians who favored the replacement of midwives with obstetric charities include the following: Greer Baughman, "A Preliminary Report Upon the Midwife Situation in Virginia," *Virginia Medical Monthly*, 54 (March 1928), 749; Henry Schwartz, "Prenatal Care," *Transactions of the American Association for the Study and Prevention of Infant Mortality*, 4 (1913), 180.

35. Ziegler, "The Elimination of the Midwife," 231; W. W. Chipman, "Teaching Obstetrics: Necessary Equipment," *Transactions of the American Association for the Study and Prevention of Infant Mortality*, 5 (1914), 184; De Lee, "Progress," 114-115; Moran, "Endowment," 125; Huntington, "The Midwife in Massachusetts," 419.

36. Edward P. Davis, "The Springs of a Nation's Life," *Transactions of the American Association for the Study and Prevention of Infant Mortality*, 9 (1918), 111.

37. Baughman, "Preliminary Report," 749; O. R. Thompson, "Midwife Problem," *Journal of the Medical Association of Georgia*, 16 (April 1927), 136. See also Helmina Jeidell and Willa M. Fricke, "The Midwives of Anne Arundel, County, Maryland," *Johns Hopkins Medical Bulletin*, 23 (1912), 279-281; W. A. Plecker, "The Midwife Problem in Virginia," *Virginia Medical Semi-Monthly*, 19 (December 1914), 456-458.

38. E. R. Hardin, "The Midwife Problem," *Southern Medical Journal*, 18 (1925), 348-349.

39. Emmons and Huntington, "Has the Trained and Supervised Midwife," 207-208; Emmons and Huntington, "A Review of the Midwife Situation," 261.

40. Arthur B. Emmons, "Obstetrics," *Transactions of the American*

Association for the Study and Prevention of Infant Mortality, 7 (1916), 39; Davis, "The Need of Hospitals," 197; James L. Huntington, "The Regulation of Midwifery," *Boston Medical and Surgical Journal*, 167 (1912), 84.

41. Ziegler, "The Elimination of the Midwife," 222-234. Ten years later Ziegler was still arguing that "it will not get us anywhere to say that midwives do just as good work as the average doctor, which may be true. It should not be a question of the lesser of two evils. Neither is fit. We want something better; we want well trained doctors to attend women in confinement." Charles E. Ziegler, "How Can We Best Solve the Midwifery Problem?," *American Journal of Public Health*, 12 (1922), 412.

42. George W. Kosmak, "Does the Average Midwife Meet the Requirements?" *Transactions of the American Association for the Study and Prevention of Infant Mortality*, 3 (1912), 250.
Curiously, the American Medical Association (AMA) did not adopt an official resolution with regard to the midwife question. This is probably related to the fact that as early as 1883 the association began to view the establishment of specialist bodies, such as the American Gynecological Society (1876), as a serious threat to its own strength. With the general reorganization of the AMA in 1901, an attempt was made to bring the specialist back into the ranks of the general medical societies. Nevertheless, the general practitioner remained the "predominant AMA voter" during the early years of the twentieth century. Susan Crawford, *Digest of Official Actions: American Medical Association, 1846-1958* ([Chicago], 1959), pp. i, 518; James G. Burrow, *AMA: Voice of American Medicine* (Baltimore, 1963), p. 7; William G. Rothstein, *American Physicians in the Nineteenth Century: From Sects to Science* (Baltimore, 1972), p. 318; Stevens, *American Medicine*, p. 124. For more information on the general practitioner-specialist conflict, see Stevens, *American Medicine*, Chapters 2, 6; Gerald E. Markowitz and David Karl Rosner, "Doctors in Crisis: A Study of the Use of Medical Education Reform to Establish Modern Professional Elitism in Medicine," *American Quarterly*, 25 (March 1973), 83-107.

43. Baldy, "Is the Midwife," 105; De Lee, "Progress," 115; Emmons and Huntington, "Has the Trained and Supervised Midwife," 208; L. R. Williams, "Position of the New York State Department of Health in Relation to the Control of Midwives," *New York State Journal of Medicine*, 15 (August 1915), 299; Ziegler, "The Elimination of the Midwife," 222.

44. "Discussion—Dr. H. W. N. Bennett," *Transactions of the American Association for the Study and Prevention of Infant Mortality*, 5 (1914), 205; Williams, "The Midwife Problem," 189.

45. William R. Nicholson, "The Midwife Situation," *Transactions of the American Gynecological Society*, 42 (1917), 623; L. R. Williams, "Position, 300; Baldy, "Is the Midwife," 108. See also Davis, "The Springs," 111.

46. De Lee, "Progress," 118.

47. Felix J. Underwood, "The Development of Midwifery in Virginia," *Southern Medical Journal*, 19 (September 1926), 683.

48. Thompson, "Midwife Problem," 136; W. A. Plecker, "The Midwife in Virginia," *Virginia Medical Semi-Monthly*, 18 (January 1914), 475.

49. See, for example, Mary Roth Walsh, *"Doctors Wanted: No Women Need Apply." Sexual Barriers in the Medical Profession, 1835-1975* (New Haven, Conn., 1977), pp. 106-206.

50. Paine, "The Midwife Problem," 760.

51. Emmons and Huntington, "Has the Trained and Supervised Midwife," 199-213; Emmons and Huntington, "A Review of the Midwife Situation," 251-262; Huntington, "The Midwife in Massachusetts," 418-421; James L. Huntington, "Midwives in Massachusetts," *Transactions of the American Association for the Study and Prevention of Infant Mortality*, 3 (1912), 266-271; James L. Huntington, "The Pregnancy Clinic and the Midwife: A Comparison," *Boston Medical and Surgical Journal*, 173 (November 1915), 764-766.

52. "Reports—New England Sub-Committee on Obstetrics," *Transactions of the American Association for the Study and Prevention of Infant Mortality*, 4 (1913), 222.

53. Other critics who demanded the immediate elimination of the midwife include the following: De Lee, "Progress," 114; Ziegler, "The Elimination of the Midwife," 223.

54. J. Clifton Edgar, "The Remedy for the Midwife Problem," *American Journal of Obstetrics and the Diseases of Women and Children*, 63 (1911), 881.

55. J. Clifton Edgar, "The Education," 92, 96-97. See also J. Clifton Edgar, "Why the Midwife?" *American Journal of Obstetrics and the Diseases of Women and Children*, 77 (1918), 243. Similar views were expressed in the following articles: Edmund F. Cody, "The Registered Midwife: A Necessity," *Boston Medical and Surgical Journal*, 168 (March 1913), 416-418; Nicholson, "The Midwife Situation," 623-631; William R. Nicholson, *An Anachronism of the Twentieth Century: The Midwife*, Nathan Lewis Hatfield Lectures [Philadelphia, 1921], pp. 3-31.

56. S. W. Newmayer, "The Status of Midwifery in Pennsylvania and a Study of the Midwives in Philadelphia," *Monthly Cyclopedia and Medical Bulletin*, 4 (1911), 713, 718.

57. For example, see notes 37, 38, this chapter.

58. Jessie L. Marriner, *Midwifery in Alabama* (Alabama State Board of Health [1925]), pp. 1-2, 10.

59. *Report*, Board of Health of Mississippi (1919-1921), p. 198.

60. Plecker, "The Midwife in Virginia," 475; Plecker, "The Midwife

Problem in Virginia," 456-458; W. A. Plecker, "The First Move Toward Midwife Control in Virginia," *Virginia Medical Monthly*, 45 (April 1918), 12-13; W. A. Plecker, "Virginia Makes Efforts to Solve Midwife Problem," *Nation's Health*, 7 (December 1925), 809-811. Other southerners who felt that the midwife was a necessary evil include the following: Paul Crumpler, "The Midwife," *Charlotte (North Carolina) Medical Journal*, 73 (1916), 159-160; Hardin, "The Midwife Problem," 347-350.

61. See, for example, Charles E. Terry, "Save the Seventh Baby," *Delineator*, 92 (October 1917), 15-16; Olivia Dunbar, "To the Baby, Debtor," *Good Housekeeping*, 67 (November 1918), 35; S. Josephine Baker, "Getting the Right Start," *Ladies' Home Journal*, 47 (August 1930), 80; Anna S. Richardson, "Safety First for Mother," *McClure's*, 45 (May 1915), 97.

62. Woods Hutchinson, "When the Stork Arrives," *Good Housekeeping*, 59 (July 1914), 102; Anna S. Richardson, "Safeguarding American Motherhood," *McClure's*, 45 (July 1915), 35.

63. Joseph B. De Lee, "Before the Baby Comes," *Delineator*, 109 (October 1926), 84. See also Mary E. Bayley, "The Prospective Mother," *Delineator*, 99 (September 1921), 30; B. Wallace Hamilton, "Before the Baby Arrives," *Delineator*, 93 (October 1918), 24; Harvey W. Wiley, "Getting Ready for Baby," *Good Housekeeping*, 74 (April 1922), 59; Frank W. Lynch, "A Child Is to Be Born," *Hygenia*, 4 (May 1926), 255; Gulielma Alsop, "The Right to Be Well Born," *Woman Citizen*, 8 (February 1924), 30.

64. Charlotte Teller, "The Neglected Psychology of the 'Twilight Sleep,'" *Good Housekeeping*, 6 (July 1915), 17; Tracy and Leupp, "Painless Childbirth," 42; Leupp and Hendrick, "Twilight Sleep," 37; "Is the Twilight Sleep Safe—For Me?" 10.

65. Charles E. Terry, "The Mother, the Midwife—and the Law," *Delineator*, 92 (February 1916), 12-13; Terry, "Save the Seventh Baby," 15-16; Carolyn C. Van Blarcom, "Rat Pie: Among the Black Midwives of the South," *Harper's*, 160 (February 1930), 322-332.

66. "Supervision of Midwives in New York City," *Weekly Bulletin*, Department of Health, City of New York, 10 (May 1921), 153; *Fifty-First Annual Report*, New Jersey State Department of Health (1928), 153; Marriner, *Midwifery*, p. 10.

6

The Early
Twentieth-Century
Midwife Debate: Proponents

Most of the support for the midwife came from public health officials who were distressed about the high infant and maternal mortality rates in the United States. They believed that the number of infant and maternal deaths would be substantially reduced if the midwife were properly trained and regulated. On numerous occasions, they defended the midwife against opponents who characterized her as "ignorant" and "dirty." As an example, Clara D. Noyes, general superintendent of training schools at the Bellevue and Allied Hospitals in New York City, read a paper before the International Congress of Hygiene and Demography in 1912 in which she argued that the American midwife should not be condemned "too harshly for her lack of training." Noyes pointed out that all too often the midwife attempted to secure an education "only to find that after spending money and time, she has been exploited and the few lectures she has heard and the pretentious diploma which she has received are of little practical value." She concluded that "it would be preposterous to expect the midwife to be other than she is" as long as the United States continued to enact so few provisions in her behalf.[1]

Other midwife proponents supported this view. For example, the commissioner of health of New York City chastised the United States for being "the only civilized country in the world in which the health as well as the life and future well-being of mothers and infants is not safeguarded so far as is possible through the training and control of midwives." Likewise, an article appearing in the *Quarterly Bulletin* of the Rhode Island State Board of Health pointed out that "we are the only country in the world without statutory legislation governing, controlling, and supervising midwives yet 40 percent of our births are attended by midwives."[2]

Midwife proponents were well aware that the maternal and infant mortality rates in most European countries were substantially lower than those in the United States. They attributed special significance to these figures because the percentage of midwife-attended births was much higher in Europe than in the United States. Proponents of the trained and regulated midwife often utilized these statistics in their attempts to convince the medical profession and the public of the need to provide comprehensive programs for the American midwife.

Carolyn C. Van Blarcom, a graduate nurse, who served as secretary of the Committee for the Prevention of Blindness for the State of New York and chairwoman of the Committee on Midwives of the National Organization for Public Health Nursing, wrote several articles and one book on this topic. She compared the situation in America with that in Denmark where 90-95 percent of all births were attended by midwives "without nearly the same high death-rate among infants."[3]

The European country with which Van Blarcom was most familiar, however, was England. After spending the autumn of 1911 studying the working of the English Midwives Act of 1902, she concluded that "the situation in England prior to 1902, when the Midwives Act became a law, closely parallelled conditions which exist in America . . . today." With the passage of the 1902 act, the English infant mortality rate was reduced from 151 deaths per 1,000 live births during 1901 to 106 deaths per 1,000 live births in 1910. Although Van Blarcom conceded that this decrease was not solely attributable to better trained midwives, she was convinced that "the better obstetrical work now being done in England must be regarded as one factor in the decreased death-rate."[4]

About 50 percent of the births in both England and the United States were attended by midwives in 1910. Nevertheless, the 1910 infant mortality rate per 1,000 live births for the United States was

124—substantially higher than the English rate of 106. Van Blarcom believed that the infant death rate in the United States could be reduced if Americans would set to work on their own midwife problem by enacting legislation similar to that adopted in England.[5]

Van Blarcom was not the only proponent who gathered information on midwife training programs in Europe. Dr. S. Josephine Baker conducted a lengthy study of European midwifery regulations which she presented to the 1911 annual meeting of the American Association for the Study and Prevention of Infant Mortality. She contrasted the methods of midwife control in the United States, which were "remarkable mainly for their deficiency," with the relatively successful programs that were established in the major countries of Europe. Baker hoped that her study would help convince the members of the AASPIM to take a more active stand in behalf of midwife education and control.[6] Most members of the association, however, were interested in reforming obstetric education and elevating the status of the obstetrician. At best, they viewed regulatory legislation as a temporary measure designed to lead to the midwife's ultimate elimination.[7]

Defenders of the midwife also publicized the fact that maternal and infant mortality rates had been significantly reduced in those few American cities and states which had adopted comprehensive training and regulatory programs for their midwives. The two locations which received the most publicity were New York City and New Jersey.

The publicity which New York City received resulted from the fact that it was the first city in the United States to establish a Bureau of Child Hygiene (1908) as well as the first city to create a municipally sponsored school for midwives (Bellevue, 1911). Moreover, it enacted some of the most comprehensive regulatory legislation of any locality in America.[8] In 1907, one year before the bureau was established, the infant mortality rate of New York City was 144 deaths per 1,000 live births. By 1921, that figure had been reduced by more than one-half to 71.1 deaths.[9] Certainly, the training and supervision of New York's midwives, who attended between 26 and 40 percent of the births in the city from 1910 to 1920, was a significant factor in bringing about this decline. In fact, a report issued by the Department of Health of New York City in 1921 stated that the regulation and supervision of midwives had "an important bearing upon the prevention of maternal and infant morbidity and mortality." The report concluded that "with better midwives, there have come better mothers, better babies, and a better infant mortality rate."[10]

S. Josephine Baker, who served with the New York City Department of Health for more than a quarter of a century, worked diligently to convince the public of the value of developing comprehensive programs for midwives. She wrote articles for medical journals and popular magazines in which she described the New York City program. Finally, in 1925, she published a book, *Child Hygiene,* which included a brief history of New York City's efforts to reduce its maternal and infant mortality rates through midwife training and control. Baker's New York City experience enabled her to develop a strong defense in behalf of the midwife which her opponents found difficult to criticize. The papers and other comments she presented to the predominantly hostile American Association for the Study and Prevention of Infant Mortality were strengthened because of her personal involvement in the New York City program.[11]

The efforts of New Jersey, and especially Newark, to train and regulate their midwives also received a good deal of publicity. Provisions for the licensing of New Jersey midwives were first made in 1892 when the State Board of Medical Examiners was given the authority to issue licenses. In 1910, the law was amended to require that the prospective midwife be a graduate of a recognized school of midwifery and satisfactorily pass an examination given by the board.[12]

Three years later, in 1913, Newark created a Division of Child Hygiene. Dr. Julius Levy, who headed the division, promptly inaugurated a series of conferences and lectures for the purpose of educating the midwife and informing her of the provisions of the 1910 law. In 1917, Levy reported that there were ninety-six practicing midwives in Newark, only two of whom were unlicensed. He commended Newark's midwives for conscientiously using silver nitrate as a prophylactic against ophthalmia neonatorum. He pointed out that there were no midwives who were known to carry drugs or surgical instruments in their bags. He also reported that most midwives promptly called a physician when abnormal symptoms were present. Levy concluded that he saw "little reason for condemnation or elimination of the midwife, or the establishment of costlier hospitals to care for all maternity cases." The Newark experiment had justified his faith in the usefulness of the midwife "under proper supervision and cooperation." Two years later, Levy concluded that the public health education which Newark midwives received each year had resulted in an additional "100 teachers of infant hygiene to our staff, and that the policy of ignoring the midwife or denying her existence helps no one—except the undertaker."[13]

Following Newark's example, New Jersey created a Bureau of Child Hygiene late in 1918. Levy was appointed its chief, and he remained in that office until his retirement in 1951.[14] One of the first projects of the newly established bureau was to conduct a statewide survey of New Jersey's midwives. The completed survey indicated that 40 percent of all births in New Jersey were attended by midwives in 1919. Unfortunately, the majority of these women were judged to be "ignorant, dirty, and negligent." Seven years later, however, Dr. Henry B. Costill, director of the New Jersey State Department of Health, was able to report that "the great majority" of New Jersey's midwives wear white sterilized gowns and caps, use boiled rubber gloves, and carry bags which are "properly supplied with clean equipment which can compare favorably with the bags carried by careful physicians."[15]

Costill attributed the success of New Jersey's program to "organization and sympathetic vigorous supervision." He congratulated Levy for his "vision and courage . . . in the face of medical opposition and without precedent as a guide." Costill was especially pleased with the work performed by New Jersey's district midwifery supervisors, who helped the midwives form their own county associations. These associations, which usually met monthly, provided New Jersey midwives with the opportunity to meet together on a regular basis and discuss their midwifery experiences. Moreover, at each meeting, physicians and nurses gave formal lectures on specific aspects of obstetrics. In 1924, eighty-three meetings were held with a total statewide attendance of 1,057. In that same year, annual statewide conferences for midwives were initiated and plans were made for a postgraduate course for midwives. The New Jersey Department of Health reported in 1926 that these "annual conferences are fostering a real pride in professional standards and are doing a great deal to place midwifery in New Jersey on the high plane that work as serious and responsible as midwifery should be."[16]

New Jersey continued to institute positive measures in behalf of its midwives throughout the remainder of the 1920s. In 1927, for example, the Bureau of Child Hygiene began publishing a quarterly bulletin, the *Progressive Midwife*. The purpose of the bulletin was "to acquaint the progressive midwives of New Jersey with the accomplishments, aims and problems of all work concerning the welfare of mothers and babies." The significance of this bulletin was underscored by the fact that New Jersey was evidently the only state to publish a magazine expressly for its midwives.[17]

The early issues of the *Progressive Midwife* were typewritten and about four to six pages in length. When it ceased publication in February 1932, the length of the bulletin had doubled. In addition, the later issues were printed on quality paper and featured photographs. The *Progressive Midwife* published educational articles on pregnancy, parturition, and postpartum care. It also carried announcements and reports of county association meetings. The editors of the magazine were proud that New Jersey required its midwives to have at least 1,800 hours of training over a nine-month period in order to qualify for a license. They published articles in which they compared New Jersey's efforts at training and regulation with the less comprehensive programs of other states.[18]

New Jersey, like New York City, experienced a drop in its maternal and infant mortality rates after its midwife program was instituted. In 1914, a few months after the Newark Division of Child Hygiene was established, Newark reported a maternal mortality rate of 5.3 per 1,000 live births. By 1916, the rate had been reduced to 2.2. Julius Levy concluded that

these figures indicate that there has been a considerable reduction of maternal mortality in the three years that the [Newark] Department of Health has maintained supervision over midwifery, and that in 1916, with approximately 50 per cent of the births attended by midwives, the rate of the city of Newark was among the lowest in the country.[19]

Levy wrote several articles in which he compared New Jersey's maternal and infant mortality rates with those of states which had not developed thoroughgoing training and regulatory programs. For example, the 1916 infant mortality rate for Newark was 89.6 per 1,000 live births, while Baltimore reported a rate of 118.1; Boston, 104; Detroit, 112.8. Levy also reported that the 1916 infant mortality rate for births attended by Newark midwives was lower (70.7) than that of Newark physicians (74.3). Furthermore, he published an article in the *American Journal of Public Health* in 1923 which indicated that maternal mortality rates were lowest in those New Jersey counties which had the highest percentage of midwife-attended births. Thus, he concluded that abolishing the midwife would not help solve the problem of the high maternal mortality rates in the United States.[20]

Several other states also made significant progress in midwife training and control. For example, the actions taken by the Connecticut Bureau of Child Hygiene closely paralleled those of the New Jersey bureau. Unlike New Jersey, however, the Connecticut program received little publicity.[21]

The first law requiring Connecticut midwives to be licensed was passed in 1893. For nine years, midwives were licensed by the Connecticut Medical Examining Board. In 1902, a special Board of Examiners in Midwifery was established. Efforts at midwife training and regulation were stepped up in 1919 with the establishment of the Connecticut Bureau of Child Hygiene. In that year, a law was passed requiring the annual registration of all licensed midwives. Three years later, the head of the Bureau of Child Hygiene appointed a state instructor of midwives who was responsible for visiting the midwives, assessing their qualifications, and organizing classes for them. A survey conducted by the instructor in 1922 indicated that there were 113 active licensed midwives in the state. Approximately 12.5 percent of all births were attended by midwives.[22]

A new midwifery law was enacted in 1923. This statute carefully specified what was and was not expected of the midwife. In the same year, the Bureau of Child Hygiene inaugurated a series of conferences for midwives which were held in various localities throughout the state. The bureau also aided the midwives of Bridgeport in forming their own association. Other local organizations were soon formed, and in 1924 the Connecticut Association of Midwives was established.[23]

Throughout the 1920s, the Connecticut Bureau of Child Hygiene, like its New Jersey counterpart, sponsored lectures, conferences, and other educational programs for its midwives. The bureau was quite pleased with the work that these women were accomplishing. In 1925, it reported that "the spirit that the midwives are showing in their work is a subject for gratification."[24]

During the late 1920s, however, the Connecticut bureau began expressing concern over the fact that many of its "good midwives" had been forced to enter other occupations because of the small number of cases available to them. By 1928, midwives attended only 8.1 percent of the births in Connecticut. The bureau attributed this decline to the following four causes: (1) immigration restriction; (2) the growing number of hospital deliveries and the feeling that this was the "American way"; (3) the increased demand for time- and pain-saving drugs; and (4) the lowering of the birth rate. In an attempt to solve the problem of the declining number of midwife-attended births, the bureau encouraged the midwives to move to rural communities that were in great need of additional medical personnel. It recognized, however, that most midwives were not able to move about freely because "nearly all are married and must stay where their husbands can get work."[25]

Health officials in New Jersey and New York City also took notice of the fact that midwives were attending fewer and fewer births. The number of midwife-attended births in New Jersey declined from 42 percent in 1918 to 19.2 percent in 1927. The New Jersey Bureau of Child Hygiene attributed part of this decline to the "raising of the standards of midwifery" and "constant supervision." The bureau quickly added, however, that "the purpose of supervision is primarily to obtain for the mothers the best possible service." It regarded the reduction in the number of cases delivered by midwives as an "indirect effect" of supervision.[26]

Similarly, the number of midwife-attended births in New York City declined from 40.35 percent in 1909 to 26.6 percent in 1920. Health officials also attributed part of this decline to New York City's rigorous training and supervision program. Nevertheless, they did not want to see the midwife completely eliminated because "every expectant mother had the right to ask, if she so desires, that she be delivered at home." They feared that eliminating the midwife would contribute to the disruption of the "cornerstone of American society"—the home. Health officials also argued that there were not enough maternity institutions and private practitioners in New York City to handle all the births presently delivered by midwives.[27]

The Bureaus of Child Hygiene of Connecticut, New Jersey, and New York City helped lead the way in midwife training and regulation. Most other cities and states were slow in adopting similar measures. In 1923, nineteen states had no definite laws and regulations governing the practices of midwives. There were no state-sponsored schools for midwives, although several states required that the midwife be a graduate of a "recognized" school. Contemporaries generally agreed that the existing schools were "more for the purpose of gain than any educational facilities that they might be supposed to offer." In addition, the laws and regulations regarding the midwife were often ignored.[28]

The impetus which eventually stimulated other states to adopt programs in behalf of their midwives came with the passage by the United States Congress of the Sheppard-Towner Maternity and Infancy Protection Act of 1921. This act provided for "instruction in the hygiene of maternity and infancy through public-health nurses, visiting nurses, consultation centers, child-care conferences, and literature distribution." The money appropriated for this program, which totaled $7,680,000 for the six-year period ending June 30, 1927, was administered by the Children's Bureau. The funds were channeled through the bureaus of child hygiene of the various states on a population percentage and matching basis. Eventually, every state except Connecticut, Illinois, and Massachusetts participated in this program.[29]

The passage of the Sheppard-Towner Act did not come about easily. The American Medical Association's fear of state-controlled medicine caused it to lobby assiduously against the proposed act. Likewise, several state medical societies also opposed it. In contrast, the Children's Bureau supported the act on the grounds that it would help eliminate the high maternal and infant mortality rates in the United States. Moreover, a powerful lobby in its support was engineered by several women's groups including the American

Medical Women's Association, the League of Women Voters, and the Women's Joint Congressional Committee. In fact, J. Stanley Lemons has concluded that the fear of being punished at the polls by newly enfranchised women played a major role in convincing politicians to support the bill.[30]

One way that Sheppard-Towner funds were utilized was to establish midwife training and regulatory programs. Dr. Anna E. Rude, director of the Maternal and Infant Hygiene Section of the Children's Bureau, reported in 1923 that money made available through the Sheppard-Towner Act had enabled thirty-one states "to attack the long neglected problem of midwife practice." For example, in 1922 the South Carolina Bureau of Child Hygiene used $20,000 of its Sheppard-Towner appropriation for midwife training and supervision. Health officials in Mississippi reported that the acceptance of the Sheppard-Towner Act had enabled that state "to devote more time and energy" to the training of its midwives. Sheppard-Towner funds also permitted the Virginia Board of Health to appoint its first supervisor of midwife education.[31]

The Sheppard-Towner Act was extended for a two-year period in 1927. By that time, however, opponents of the act had gathered enough support to force the proponents to agree to a compromise which repealed the law when it expired on June 30, 1929. Congress, which was no longer worried about a women's voting bloc, heeded the demands of the powerful American Medical Association.[32]

State health officials expressed dismay and bewilderment when the act was allowed to expire. The director of the Division of Child Hygiene of the Georgia State Board of Health wrote that the anticipated withdrawal of Sheppard-Towner funds in June 1929 posed a "serious" problem with regard to midwife training and regulation. He was quite "anxious to find some [other] way in which the instruction of midwives" could be carried out. He suggested that perhaps each county medical society could secure a physician to be responsible for training and supervising the midwives of his county. Similarly, South Carolina reported that the cutting off of Sheppard-Towner funds forced a "drastic" curtailment of its midwife staff.[33]

Actually, however, the Sheppard-Towner appropriation was quite small. The act authorized $1,240,000 in federal funds for maternal and child hygiene during the fiscal year 1922-1923. In contrast, England spent $8,638,315 toward proper prenatal care during the same period.[34] Nevertheless, the expiration of the act resulted in states throughout the nation restricting their maternal and infant hygiene programs. With the deepening of the depression, several states were even forced to drop their programs. Federal support for maternal and child health care was not reestablished until the enactment of the Social Security Act of 1935.[35]

The recognition that the maternal and infant mortality rates in the United States were excessively high was primarily responsible for convincing public health officials to work for midwife training and regulatory programs. There were other public health problems, however, which were integrally related to the midwife question. One such problem was the high rate of blindness resulting from ophthalmia neonatorum.

Blindness from "babies' sore eyes," as the disease was often called, was almost 100 percent preventable if the newborn infant's eyes were properly treated with a silver nitrate solution immediately after birth. Unfortunately, many midwives were unaware of this procedure; others were prevented by law from using any drugs, including silver nitrate. In Illinois, for example, the midwife had the choice of breaking the law or leaving the baby's eyes to chance. Dr. Caroline Hedger presented a paper to the South Side Branch of the Chicago Medical Society in 1912 in which she elaborated on this dilemma. She urged the Chicago doctors to support legislation which not only permitted but demanded "that a prophylactic be used by midwives and that every midwife be thoroughly and personally instructed as to proper methods."[36]

Similarly, Hiram Woods, a Baltimore physician, expressed concern about the increasing number of cases of ophthalmia neonatorum occurring in Maryland. He urged the Medical and Chirurgical Faculty of Maryland and the Maryland Society for Prevention of Blindness to work with the state health department in teaching midwives how to use the silver nitrate solution. He estimated that "patience, cleanliness and the use of the proper remedy will cure 98 out of 100" cases.[37]

The organization which was apparently most concerned about the relationship between poor midwife training and the high rate of ophthalmia neonatorum was the Committee for Prevention of Blindness of the State of New York. The committee estimated in 1913 that 10,000 people in the United States suffered from blindness due to ophthalmia neonatorum. Further investigations showed that much of this blindness was the result of work done by "ignorant and untrained" midwives. Following this disclosure, the committee conducted a study of midwifery conditions in fourteen European countries and Australia in order to determine how other nations dealt with their midwives and what the results of training and supervision were "when measured in the terms of the health of mothers and babies." Upon the completion of the study, the committee concluded that "the present needs in America are more nearly met by the system obtaining in England than in any other country." It published a book on the working of the English Midwives Act of 1902 and urged the United States to enact similar legislation. Thus, the committee's efforts to reduce the number of cases of ophthalmia neonatorum caused it to become actively involved in the campaign for the better training and regulation of midwives.[38]

While most physicians expressed opposition to the midwife, some members of the medical profession spoke out in her behalf. Several doctors, in fact, were quite disturbed about the opposition emanating from the medical profession. For example, in 1905, Dr. Guy Steele of Cambridge, Maryland, urged his fellow physicians to join him in supporting the educated and licensed midwife. He argued that it did not matter that this might result in "legislating fees out of our own pockets . . . [because] it has been the glory of medicine that every advance in scientific discovery, every improvement in surgical technique, has been made solely with the purpose of better serving and better helping our fellow-man." In a somewhat more critical tone, Walter H. Allport, a Chicago physician, declared:

The midwife of the present day has been so scared by the noise made by her male competitor in his efforts to accomplish her annihilation, or to bring her, at least, to a proper sense of her true and very humble position as a subordinate handmaid of science, that her voice is now seldom heard in her own defense.[39]

Significantly, the American Medical Association (AMA) never adopted an official resolution with regard to the midwife question.[40]

The articles on the midwife which appeared in the *Journal of the American Medical Association* between 1900 and 1930 often reflected opposing viewpoints. Moreover, no one opinion prevailed. About an equal number of articles and abstracts in support of and in opposition to the midwife were published during this period.[41]

Perhaps the ambivalence of the AMA toward the midwife was related to the fact that the general practitioner, rather than the specialist, was the "predominant AMA voter" during the early years of the twentieth century. Many general practitioners felt threatened by the rapid growth of specialist bodies, such as the American Gynecological Society (1876) and the American Association of Obstetricians and Gynecologists (1888). They may have feared that the adoption of an anti-midwife resolution would have bolstered the position of those physicians who argued that obstetrics was, indeed, a complicated medical specialty. Besides, many of the criticisms which the specialists heaped upon the midwife were also directed toward the general practitioner.[42]

T. J. Hill, a New York physician and midwife proponent, succinctly described the general practitioner-specialist controversy in an article published in *Medical Record* in 1898. He argued that by

suppressing the midwife we open wide the gates to our professional sisters and flood the whole country with female doctors. Practically, we hand this individual over [*sic*] the family practice, for between her and the specialist, whom she greatly admires, there will be no room for the general practitioner; he will get squeezed between the millstones.

By contrast, Hill believed that the midwife could be taught to "listen eagerly" to the male physician. "She [midwife] will sit at the feet of her Gamaliel," remarked Hill, "and hearken to his admonitions on things pertaining to the art of obstetrics."[43]

A few prominent physicians were, in fact, staunch supporters of the trained and regulated midwife. For example, Abraham Jacobi, a distinguished American pediatrician who was elected president of the American Medical Association in 1912, defended the midwife in both his opening and farewell addresses to the AMA. He sharply criticized the medical profession and the public for ignoring the needs of the midwife. "Where," he asked, "are the 108 schools which little Great Britain deems—on account of their scant number—insufficient for her urgent needs . . . ?" He urged the members of the association to support both the training and registration of midwives. Like many other midwife proponents, he argued that it was "ludicrous" to oppose the midwife on the grounds that she competed with the physician. He wanted competent midwives to attend normal births in order that doctors might be freed to learn more about abnormal and complicated pregnancies.[44]

Less well-known physicians also supported the concept of the trained and regulated midwife. The success of the midwife programs in Connecticut and New Jersey was, at least, partially attributable to the assistance received from local physicians. Doctors in both states cooperated with midwife officials by presenting lectures and demonstrations at the meetings of local midwife associations. Further evidence of medical support for the midwife is demonstrated by the fact that Connecticut held its statewide midwife institutes in large urban hospitals. Similarly, New Jersey usually conducted its annual conference for midwives at the Academy of Medicine in Newark. The New Jersey Bureau of Child Hygiene noted in 1928 that "this fact alone, indicates the progress the midwives have made and the great improvement that has taken place in the relationship which exists between the midwives and the nurses and the doctors."[45]

Physicians in Georgia also supported the concept of the trained and regulated midwife. In fact, the Medical Association of Georgia was one of the first organizations in that state to recognize the need for a comprehensive midwife program. On May 9, 1924, it passed a resolution which recommended that the

State Board of Health be requested to give such [midwife] instruction and regulations as they think best, and that this instruction be given under the supervision and direction of some physician who is a member of this Association, in each county, and if such membership is not represented, some ethical physician in each county.[46]

The following year, the Georgia State Board of Health set forth the regulations governing the practices of midwives. The regulations prescribed that each prospective midwife attend a series of ten lessons and satisfactorily pass an examination before qualifying for certification. Most midwife instruction was conducted by itinerant nurses. The Georgia State Board of Health reported in 1932, however, that "many of the doctors have continued their assistance by giving instruction to the midwives who failed to secure a certificate, inspecting their bags, and vaccinating them against smallpox after the nurse left the county. . . ."[47]

It is interesting to speculate why physicians in Georgia took the initiative in establishing a training and regulatory program for midwives. Certainly, the low economic level of the midwife and her patients caused doctors to realize that they would gain little, if any, profit by assuming the cases attended by midwives. The Georgia State Board of Health reported in 1932 that the economic condition of many midwives was so "deplorable" that they could not collect for their service and, consequently, could not buy the necessary equipment for their bags. In addition, the rural sections of Georgia were in great need of additional physicians. In 1928, the director of the Georgia Bureau of Child Hygiene pointed out that there were several counties which had no physicians and that the country doctor served an average of 1,402 people. Many Georgia doctors already had too much work to perform without taking on additional cases. They would have encountered numerous problems and hardships if they had also been obliged to look after the 31.4 percent of births attended by Georgia midwives in 1927.[48]

Significantly, women physicians who were not actively involved in public health programs tended to remain aloof from the midwife debate. The concern which Dr. S. Josephine Baker voiced for the midwife was not indicative of the sentiment expressed by most other female medical practitioners. Articles published in the *Medical Woman's Journal* (formerly the *Woman's Medical Journal*), probably the most important periodical published expressly for women physicians during this period, had very little to say about the midwife. While several of the articles published in the journal supported the view that the status of obstetrics needed to be improved, the authors did not comment on whether they believed that eliminating the midwife would help achieve this goal. Even articles on America's high infant and maternal mortality rates did not usually discuss the midwife. Rather, they emphasized the need for pure milk, better vital statistics, and proper prenatal care. Moreover, very few of the midwife articles published in the standard medical journals of the period were written by women physicians.

At least one female practitioner did argue, however, that the woman doctor made a better birth attendant than either the midwife or the male doctor.[49]

Midwives, unlike physicians, did not often have the opportunity to defend themselves publicly against the attacks of their opponents. They faced the serious problem of having few organizations and publications through which their voices might be heard. Only two periodicals were discovered for the 1900-1930 period which were written expressly for American midwives. The first of these publications was a short-lived bulletin entitled *Topics of Interest to Midwives*. It was published by a Chicago physician, Ferdinand Herb, on a monthly basis during 1918. The bulletin was sent free of charge to the midwives of Chicago. Herb was disturbed that "the usual avenues of advancement to progress are practically closed to midwives." Thus, he began editing *Topics of Interest to Midwives* in order "to furnish to the ambitious midwife the lacking opportunity to keep up with the progress of the times." Each issue of the bulletin contained a simple lesson relating to pregnancy and motherhood.[50]

No other magazine for midwives was published until the New Jersey Bureau of Child Hygiene began issuing the *Progressive Midwife* in 1927. Although it remained in existence until 1932, the *Progressive Midwife*, like *Topics of Interest to Midwives*, was a local publication which reached only a select number of women. There was no national journal for midwives published during the 1900-1930 era. Midwives had to rely on nurses, public health advocates, and concerned physicians to publish articles in their behalf in the standard medical and nursing journals of the period.[51]

Similarly, attempts at organizing midwives met with only limited success during this period. The Connecticut Bureau of Child Hygiene discussed this problem in its 1929 annual report. It pointed out that Connecticut midwives preferred to work alone and that they were widely separated from each other. In an attempt to encourage midwives to participate in the activities of their local associations, the Connecticut bureau offered a banner to the best-functioning organization. The bureau reported, however, that only the Bridgeport Association had entered the competition. An anonymous article appearing in the *American Journal of Nursing* in 1926 also discussed this problem. The author called attention to the fact that there was no national lobbying agent for American midwives, such as the Midwives Institute in England. Except for the efforts of a few bureaus of child hygiene to establish educational associations for midwives, little organizational work was undertaken during this period. Indeed, most midwives remained isolated from each other between 1900 and 1930.[52]

There were no regional or national organizations for midwives during this period. It would have been very difficult to unite black "grannies" of the South with poor immigrant midwives of the urban Northeast. The language barrier, alone, posed numerous problems. Also the poor economic status of most of these women prohibited them from attending regional or national meetings. For example, the New Jersey Department of Health reported that many of the 200 midwives who attended the 1926 annual midwifery conference at the Newark Academy of Medicine "came at a great personal sacrifice of effort and money."[53] In addition, midwives who only occasionally aided a parturient friend or relative were probably reluctant to commit their time to clubs and professional associations.[54]

Because midwives were poorly organized, they were not able to help draft the laws and regulations governing their practices. For example, no statements by midwives were made before the 1927 United States Senate subcommittee hearings on the practice of medicine and midwifery in the District of Columbia. In contrast, lengthy testimony was presented by members of the recognized medical profession, as well as by representatives of the osteopaths, Christian Scientists, and optometrists.[55]

The absence of professional midwife associations was all the more significant since physicians' organizations became increasingly powerful as the twentieth century progressed. At a time when "medicine was becoming an institutionalized, collective occupation," midwives continued to go their separate and isolated ways. Specialization, group practice, and hospital affiliation provided physicians with a tremendous amount of power and influence.[56] Midwives, however, were ill-equipped to make their voices heard.

Many problems with regard to midwife training and regulation remained unsolved in 1930. The health departments of ten states reported that their midwives were neither controlled nor licensed.

Six other states indicated that they required their midwives to be registered, but not licensed. Moreover, many of the existing midwifery laws were unenforceable. The Bellevue School for Midwives was still in operation, but it was forced to close its doors in 1935 because of a lack of students. Only one other midwifery school of quality had been established. It was founded in 1923 as an affiliate of the Preston Retreat Hospital in Philadelphia. After 1930, however, few students enrolled in the Philadelphia school. In addition, the expiration of the Sheppard-Towner Act was largely responsible for the curtailment of child hygiene activities in twenty-five states between 1925 and 1930.[57]

At the same time, the maternal and infant mortality rates in the United States remained alarmingly high. Although the infant mortality rate dropped from 124 deaths per 1,000 live births in 1910 to 65 in 1930, the decline in the number of neonatal deaths (infants under one month old) was much less pronounced. This disclosure was all the more depressing since the 1930 White House Conference on Child Health and Protection estimated that neonatal deaths accounted for one-half of all infant deaths under one year. Statistics relating to maternal mortality were even more discouraging. The maternal mortality rate of the United States increased from 61 deaths per 10,000 live births in 1915 to 70 deaths in 1929.[58]

In an attempt to solve the problem of the persisting high infant and maternal mortality rates in the United States, three separate organizations engaged in exhaustive studies of the practices of midwives and physicians during the early 1930s. These studies not only examined the type of training that midwives and physicians received, but they also attempted to determine whether mortality rates were higher among births attended by midwives or physicians.

The most detailed investigation of this type was conducted by the 1930 White House Conference on Child Health and Protection. This conference, which was assembled by President Herbert Hoover in November 1930, was attended by over 3,000 people. For sixteen months prior to the conference, 1,200 experts were involved in preparatory research and study. Two of the volumes published by the conference dealt specifically with maternal and infant health care.[59]

The first of the two volumes to be published was *Obstetric Education* (1932). This lengthy work, compiled by the conference's subcommittee on obstetric teaching and education, evaluated the obstetric training of physicians, nurses, midwives, and the laity. It was highly critical of the type of obstetric education which physicians received. The report maintained that "the majority of students at the time of graduation are not qualified to assume the responsibilities of caring for maternity cases. . . . Less than half of the students have delivered any woman up to the time of graduation." The report also pointed out that midwife education left much to be desired. The methods of licensing and controlling varied from state to state and, often, midwifery laws were unenforceable. Although the subcommittee recommended that "recognized institutions for the training of midwives" be established, it believed that "the ultimate solution of the problem of good obstetrics is in developing a sufficient number of physicians who are well trained in the fundamental principle of obstetrics." Nevertheless, the subcommittee did point out, through statistical analysis, that the midwife was not "the determining factor in the high maternal mortality of any particular area" in the United States.[60]

In a supplementary report, Dr. J. H. Mason Knox, chief of the Maryland State Bureau of Child Hygiene, argued that at the international level there was a definite relationship between low maternal mortality and high percentages of births attended by midwives. He stated that it was "a little presumptuous for even well-qualified obstetricians to condemn midwives in general when our experience the world over is that in those countries in which midwives play the largest part in obstetric practice there is the lowest maternal mortality."[61]

A second volume issued by the 1930 White House Conference on Child Health and Protection, entitled *Fetal, Newborn, and Maternal Morbidity and Mortality* (1933), left little doubt as to who was responsible for the high infant and maternal mortality rates in the United States. The report concluded that "it seems possible that all the advances in medical knowledge have been almost lost to the parturient woman through too great a recourse to instrumental delivery" by the physician. One contributor to the study, Dr. E. D. Plass of Iowa City, suggested that the increase in operative deliveries, especially the forceps and cesarean sections, during the past fifteen years "may well be responsible for our failure to make any progress in the fight against the deplorable loss of life among mothers and newborn infants." The report compared the operative rate for confinements in the Scandinavian countries and England, which amounted to 15 percent, with that of the United States, which ranged from 65 to 80 percent. It also discussed some of the disadvantages of hospital deliveries including the "exposure to cross infection" and the "often false feeling of security of the operating room." The report concluded that this latter factor "undeniably has led to much unnecessary operating with its resulting trauma and increased morbidity and mortality."[62]

A second organization to make a significant investigation into the practices of midwives was the Committee on the Costs of Medical Care. This committee, created in May 1927 by fifteen leaders in the fields of medicine, public health, and the social sciences, was especially concerned about the poor quality of medical services in America. It initiated a five-year study of research in order that "the people of every locality can attack the perplexing problem of providing adequate medical care for all persons at costs within their means."[63]

The final report of the committee was published in 1932. It recommended that "unqualified 'cult' practitioners should be eliminated, and control should be exercised over the practice of secondary practitioners, such as midwives, chiropodists, and optometrists." The committee also authorized a special investigation of "secondary practitioners," which was published under the title, *Midwives, Chiropodists and Optometrists: Their Place in Medical Care* (1932).[64]

The Committee on the Costs of Medical Care estimated that there were approximately 47,000 midwives who attended 15 percent of all births in the United States in 1925. It concurred with the White House Conference on Child Health and Protection that American midwives were both poorly trained and regulated. It also disclosed that the "midwife is not the determining factor in the country's high maternal mortality rate. . . ." In fact, it maintained "that untrained midwives approach, and trained midwives surpass, the record of physicians *in normal deliveries*. . . ." The committee argued that the midwife took better care of her patients because "she waits patiently and lets nature take its course." In contrast, it accused physicians of employing "procedures which are calculated to hasten delivery, but which sometimes result harmfully to mother and child." Nevertheless, the report concluded that "it is both undesirable and unlikely that the midwife as she is generally known in the United States today should have a permanent place in medical care in this country." The committee did concede that a place might exist for the type of trained midwife found in Europe and England.[65]

The organization which was responsible for producing the most widely publicized report on the practices of midwives and physicians was the New York Academy of Medicine's Committee on Public Health Relations. Like many other groups, the New York Academy of Medicine was disturbed about the high maternal mortality rates in the United States. In New York City, for example, the maternal mortality rate increased from 5.33 maternal deaths per 1,000 live births in 1920 to 5.69 in 1932. In an attempt to discover why the maternal death rate was so high, the New York Academy of Medicine commissioned its Public Health Relations Committee to conduct a study of the causes of maternal deaths in New York City for a three-year period beginning in January 1930.[66]

The committee reported that almost 66 percent of the 2,041 maternal deaths that occurred between 1930 and 1933 were preventable. The marked incidence of operative interference was judged to be a major cause of the high maternal death rate. The committee estimated that physicians were responsible for 61.1 percent of the preventable deaths while only 2.2 percent of the deaths were attributed to the errors of midwives. The remainder of the deaths were ascribed to the poor judgment of the patients.[67]

The committee also reported that midwives had the lowest maternal death rate of any birth attendant. The maternal death rate for obstetricians, who presumably handled the more difficult cases, was 5.4 per 1,000 live births, while surgeons had a rate of 9.9. The comparable figure for midwives was 1.4. Thus, the committee concluded that "the midwife is an acceptable attendant for properly selected cases of labor and delivery. . . . We have seen that her results are as good as those obtained by the physicians under what are justly regarded as comparable circumstances for comparable cases." Interestingly, Dr. George W. Kosmak, who twenty years earlier had written articles in opposition to the midwife, served as an obstetric advisor for this study.[68]

The New York Academy of Medicine's Committee on Public Health Relations was also critical of the increased incidence of hospital deliveries. It reported that "the great increase in the hospitalization for the normal patient has failed to bring the hoped for reduction in puerperal morbidity and mortality, and this in spite of great advances in our knowledge of the processes involved and the proper way of treating them." It urged that a "program looking toward an increase in the practice of domiciliary obstetrics" be carefully investigated.[69]

The results of the New York Academy of Medicine's study were published in newspapers and magazines throughout the United States. Over 300 newspapers in thirty-nine states gave coverage to the study. Hospital committees were formed to investigate the cause of each maternal death. People throughout the country were shocked that so many pregnant women were needlessly dying. The *Nation* magazine stated: "When a doctor attacks another doctor— it is time for the general public to take notice. . . . The lay public can only hope that the figures of the future will be equally heartening after this campaign of education has got under way." In addition, the Philadelphia County Medical Society was prompted to conduct a similar investigation of maternal deaths in Philadelphia. It concluded that 56.7 percent of the 717 maternal deaths for the 1931-1933 period were preventable.[70]

Not all physicians reacted favorably to the findings of the New York Academy of Medicine. The New York Obstetrical Society issued a report in 1934 which was harshly critical of the academy's study. The New York Obstetrical Society argued that it was more correct to say that the high maternal mortality rate was due to "controllable causes" rather than that such deaths were "preventable." It disagreed with the academy's conclusion that the midwife was an acceptable birth attendant. The society maintained that "the practice of Obstetrics will never be elevated to the position it rightly deserves as long as the midwife is permitted to practice." Moreover, it condemned midwives for frequently being "a menace to the health of the women under their supervision."[71]

Three years later, Iago Galdston, the secretary on medical information for the New York Academy of Medicine, issued a rebuttal to the New York Obstetrical Society's report. Galdston included information from the Philadelphia County Medical Society's study. He also reiterated that the frequent use of forceps, anesthesia, and surgery during childbirth was a major cause of needless maternal deaths.[72]

Public health advocates were unsuccessful in their attempts to convince the medical profession and lay people that the utilization of properly trained and regulated midwives would help reduce the maternal and infant mortality rates in the United States. The number of midwife-attended births continued to decline despite the findings of powerful and influential organizations, such as the White House Conference on Child Health and Protection, the Committee on the Costs of Medical Care, and the New York Academy of Medicine. The failure of the proponents was partially attributable to the fact that their opponents were better organized and more articulate. However, social and cultural changes, only peripherally related to the early twentieth-century midwife debate, also helped to bring about the midwife's downfall.

For example, the halting of the flow of immigrants during the 1920s resulted in fewer women demanding the services of the midwife. The immigration restriction laws of 1921 and 1924 "meant that in a generation the foreign-born would cease to be a major factor in American history." By 1930, in fact, 80 percent of all practicing midwives lived in the South. Contemporary observers concurred in the opinion that immigration restriction had resulted in fewer births being attended by midwives. Health officials in Connecticut, New Jersey, and New York City, three localities heavily populated by immigrants, pointed out that the reduction in the percentage of women delivered by midwives was a result, in part, of restricted immigration. In addition, as immigrant women became "Americanized," they preferred to have their babies in hospitals under the care of specially trained physicians.[73]

The decline in the birth rate also contributed to the reduction of the number of deliveries attended by midwives. The United States experienced its "first sustained decline in the absolute number of annual births . . . between 1921 and 1933." Much of this decline was prompted by desires for higher levels of living. As the nation became increasingly urbanized and industrialized, children were no longer looked upon as assets to the household economy. Moreover, the actual cost of having a baby increased from $15 to $50 at the end of the nineteenth century to as much as $500 to $1,500 by the mid-1920s.[74]

As increasing numbers of Americans chose to have fewer children, attitudes about childbirth also changed. Birth was no longer looked upon as a routine matter. Rather, the birth of a baby was deemed a very special event which was to be planned for carefully. In addition, it was easy to juxtapose this attitude with the view that childbirth was a complex medical disorder requiring the services of the highly trained medical practitioner. Young couples often sought out the best medical help they could attain. This frequently meant entering one of the growing number of hospitals where parturient women were attended by specially trained obstetricians. Moreover, the development of the automobile provided pregnant women with a quick and easy mode of transportation to the hospital. Finally, many young women welcomed the rest from household chores which accompanied hospital confinements.[75]

In 1930, the midwife attended only 15 percent of all births in the United States. Over the succeeding years her numbers continued to decline. By 1973, for example, 99.3 percent of all births were delivered by physicians in hospitals.[76] The American midwife, who seven decades earlier had attended one-half of all births, appeared to be defeated.

NOTES

1. Clara D. Noyes, "The Training of Midwives in Relation to the Prevention of Infant Mortality," *American Journal of Obstetrics and the Diseases of Women and Children*, 66 (1912), 1056. See also Clara D. Noyes, "The Midwifery Problem," *American Journal of Nursing*, 12 (March 1912), 468. Both the *American Journal of Nursing* and the *Public Health Nurse* published a variety of articles on the need to establish training and regulatory programs for lay midwives. See, for example, Blanche F. Seyfert, "The Midwife: Her Work and the Need for Her Inspection and Instruction," *American Journal of Nursing*, 23 (April 1923), 548-550; Katherine Hagquist, "The Midwife in Texas," *Public Health Nurse*, 17 (December 1925), 612-614; Florence Swift-Wright, "Should Midwives Be Supervised by the State?" *Public Health Nurse*, 11 (1919), 413-418; Florence Swift-Wright, "Constructive Supervision of Midwives," *Public Health Nurse*, 12 (1920), 121-126.

2. Thomas Darlington, "The Present Status of the Midwife," *American Journal of Obstetrics and the Diseases of Women and Children*, 63 (1911), 871; Ira D. Hashbrouck, "Baby Week Campaign," *Quarterly Bulletin*, Rhode Island State Board of Health, 11 (April 1916), 14. See also S. Josephine Baker, "The Function of the Midwife," *Woman's Medical Journal*, 23 (September 1913), 196; Ira S. Wile, "Schools for Midwives," *Medical*

Record, 81 (March 1912), 517; Robert M. Woodbury, *Maternal Mortality: The Risk of Death in Childbirth and From All Diseases Caused by Pregnancy and Confinement*, United States Department of Labor, Children's Bureau Publication, No. 158 (Washington, D.C., 1926), p. 76.

3. Carolyn C. Van Blarcom, "Midwives in America," *American Journal of Public Health*, 4 (March 1914), 197.

4. Carolyn Conant Van Blarcom, *The Midwife in England: Being a Study in England of the Working of the English Midwives Act of 1902* (Philadelphia, 1913), p. 10. See also Carolyn C. Van Blarcom, "A Possible Solution of the Midwife Problem," *Proceedings of the National Conference of Charities and Correction*, (1910), 354; Carolyn C. Van Blarcom, "Has the Nursing Profession a Responsibility in Connection with Midwives?" *British Journal of Nursing*, 74 (September 1926), 213-214.

5. Van Blarcom, *The Midwife in England*, p. 10; Van Blarcom, "A Possible Solution," 354; Van Blarcom, "Has the Nursing Profession a Responsibility?" 213-214. For a similar opinion, see Mary Beard, "Midwifery in England," *Public Health Nursing*, 18 (1926), 634-640.

6. S. Josephine Baker, "Schools for Midwives," *Transactions of the American Association for the Study and Prevention of Infant Mortality*, 2 (1911), 233-234, passim.

7. See, for example, Joseph B. De Lee, "Progress Toward Ideal Obstetrics," *Transactions of the American Association for the Study and Prevention of Infant Mortality*, 6 (1915), 114-123; Charles E. Ziegler, "The Elimination of the Midwife," *Transactions of the American Association for the Study and Prevention of Infant Mortality*, 3 (1912), 222-237.

8. For a more detailed account of New York City's early efforts at midwife training and control, see Chapter 4, pages 51-53, of this work.

9. "One of the World's Great Citizens," *Medical Woman's Journal*, 29 (August 1922), 180-181.

10. "Supervision of Midwives in New York City," *Weekly Bulletin*, Department of Health, City of New York, 10 (May 1921), 153, 157. The report also stated that

despite the comparatively large number of infants brought into the world here by midwives during the past ten years, New York City is one of the few large cities of the country in which the maternal death rate from puerperal sepsis, and other conditions incident to pregnancy, has declined during the last decade. In other words, in the prevention of suppurative eye conditions, in maternal mortality from sepsis, and other conditions incident to pregnancy, in the number of stillbirths, in the number of deaths during the first month of life, and in the prompt reporting of births and stillbirths, the midwife, in proportion to the number of mothers delivered by her, stands on the credit side of the ledger as compared with physicians in this city. (156-157)

See also "Maternal Mortality in New York City," *Weekly Bulletin*, Department of Health, City of New York, 10 (May 1921), 170-171.

11. Baker, "The Function of the Midwife," 196-197; S. Josephine Baker, "Why Do Our Mothers and Babies Die?" *Ladies' Home Journal*, 39 (April 1922), 39, 174; S. Josephine Baker, *Child Hygiene* (New York, 1925), pp. 118-120, 488-495; Baker, "Schools for Midwives," 232-243; "Discussion," *Transactions of the American Association for the Study and Prevention of Infant Mortality*, 2 (1912), 253-255.

12. Swift-Wright, "Should Midwives Be Supervised by the State?" 416; "To Become a Licensed Registered Midwife in New Jersey," *Progressive Midwife*, 11 (February 1930), 1.

13. Stuart Galishoff, *Safeguarding the Public Health: Newark, 1895-1918* (Westport, Conn., 1975), pp. 112-113; Julius Levy, "The Maternal and Infant Mortality in Midwifery Practice in Newark, New Jersey," *American Journal of Obstetrics and the Diseases of Women and Children*, 77 (1918), 46, 49, 50-51, 53; Julius Levy, "Reduction of Infant Mortality by Economic Adjustment and by Health Education," *American Journal of Public Health*, 9 (1919), 68. See also "Midwife Supervision and Child Saving," *Survey*, 40 (August 1918), 566-567.

14. David L. Cowen, *Medicine and Health in New Jersey: A History* (Princeton, N.J., 1964), pp. 171-172.

15. Swift-Wright, "Should Midwives Be Supervised by the State?" 416; Henry B. Costill, "Midwifery Supervision Succeeds in New Jersey," *Nation's Health*, 8 (April 1926), 255, 256.

16. Costill, "Midwifery Supervision," 256, 257; "Fourth Annual Conference Notes," *Progressive Midwife*, 2 (August 1927), 2; "Cooperation and Organization Count," *Progressive Midwife*, 2 (August 1927), 4; *Forty-Ninth Annual Report*, New Jersey State Department of Health (1926), 102.

17. "Purpose," *Progressive Midwife*, 2 (August 1927), 1.

18. See, for example, "A Brief History of Obstetrics," *Progessive Midwife*, 9 (August 1929), 9; "To Become a Licensed Registered Midwife in New Jersey," 1.

19. Levy pointed out that Boston, where the midwife was outlawed, had a maternal mortality rate of 6.5 in 1916. Other cities with high maternal mortality rates in 1916 were Baltimore, 6.8; Philadelphia, 7.0. Levy, "The Maternal and Infant Mortality," 42.

20. Ibid., 43; Julius Levy, "Maternal Morbidity and Mortality in the First Month of Life in Relation to Attendant at Birth," *American Journal of Public Health*, 13 (February 1923), 90-91, 95. S. Josephine Baker published a similar article in the *Journal of the American Medical Association* in which she concluded that "comparative data do not show that the midwife can be held responsible as a dominant factor in the present high maternal

mortality rate." S. Josephine Baker, "Maternal Mortality in the United States," *Journal of the American Medical Association*, 89 (December 1927), 2017. For a rebuttal to Levy, see M. Pierce Rucker, "The Relation of the Midwife to Obstetric Mortality with Especial Reference to New Jersey," *American Journal of Public Health*, 13 (October 1923), 816-822.

21. See also Mary Evelyn Leith, "The Development of Midwife Education in South Carolina, 1919-1946" (unpublished M.A. thesis, Yale University, 1948).

22. *Thirty-Seventh Report*, Connecticut State Department of Health (1922), pp. 371, 377; *Thirty-Eighth Report*, Connecticut State Department of Health (1923), pp. 258, 264.

23. *Thirty-Eighth Report*, Connecticut State Department of Health (1923), pp. 259, 260-264; *Fortieth Report*, Connecticut State Department of Health (1925), p. 330.

24. *Fortieth Report*, Connecticut State Department of Health (1925), p. 328.

25. *Forty-Fourth Report*, Connecticut State Department of Health (1929), pp. 387, 389; *Forty-Fifth Report*, Connecticut State Department of Health (1930), p. 451.

26. *Fifty-First Annual Report*, New Jersey State Department of Health (1928), p. 153.

27. "Supervision of Midwives in New York City," 153, 154-155; "Discussion," *Transactions of the American Child Hygiene Association*, 10 (1919), 83-84.

28. Baker, *Child Hygiene*, p. 116.

29. J. Stanley Lemons, *The Woman Citizen: Social Feminism in the 1920's* (Urbana, Ill., 1973), pp. 158-159, 169; J. Stanley Lemons, "The Sheppard-Towner Act: Progressivism in the 1920's," *Journal of American History*, 55 (March 1969), 776-786; Louis S. Reed, *Midwives, Chiropodists, and Optometrists: Their Place in Medical Care* (Chicago, 1932), p. 14.

30. Lemons, *The Woman Citizen*, pp. 154-155, 162-163, 166-169; Anna E. Rude, *The Sheppard-Towner Act in Relation to Public Health* (Washington, D.C., 1922), pp. 1-8.

31. Anna E. Rude, "The Midwife Problem in the United States," *Journal of the American Medical Association*, 8 (September 1923), 989-990; Leith, "Development of Midwife Education," p. 5; Felix J. Underwood, "The Development of Midwifery in Mississippi," *Southern Medical Journal*, 19 (September 1926), 683; Emily W. Bennett, "Midwife Work in Virginia," *Public Health Nurse*, 17 (October 1925), 324. See also Azelie Ziegler, "The Midwife in the Past," *Quarterly Bulletin*, Louisiana Department of Health, 40 (September 1949), 7-8.

32. Lemons, *The Woman Citizen*, pp. 172-176.

33. Joe P. Bowdoin, "The Midwife Problem," *Transactions of the Section on Preventive Medicine and Public Health of the American Medical Association* (1928), 94; Leith, "Development of Midwife Education," pp. 9-10.

34. Matthias Nicole, "Maternity as a Public Health Problem," *American Journal of Public Health*, 19 (September 1929), 962; "Lack of Care of American Mothers," *American Journal of Nursing*, 26 (April 1926), 297.

35. Lemons, *The Woman Citizen*, pp. 175-176.

36. Caroline Hedger, "Midwives and Blindness," *Illinois Medical Journal*, 21 (April 1912), 419, 424.

37. Hiram Woods, "Professional Significance of the Midwife and Optometry Bills Passed by the Recent Legislature of Maryland," *Maryland Medical Journal*, 53 (June 1910), 189-191.

38. Van Blarcom, *The Midwife in England*, pp. 9-10.

39. Guy Steele, "The Midwife Problem and Its Legal Control," *Maryland Medical Journal*, 48 (January 1905), 2; Walter H. Allport, "Relation of the Community to the Midwife," *Chicago Medical Recorder*, 34 (1912), 124.

40. Susan Crawford, *Digest of Official Actions: American Medical Association, 1846-1958* ([Chicago], 1959), pp. i, 518.

41. See, for example, Charles E. Ziegler, "The Elimination of the Midwife," *Journal of the American Medical Association*, 60 (January 1913), 32-38; Baker, "Maternal Mortality in the United States," 2016-2017.

42. James G. Burrow, *AMA: Voice of American Medicine* (Baltimore, 1963), p. 7; William G. Rothstein, *American Physicians in the Nineteenth Century: From Sects to Science* (Baltimore, 1972), p. 318; Rosemary Stevens, *American Medicine and the Public Interest* (New Haven, Conn., 1971), p. 124. For more information on the general practitioner-specialist controversy, see Stevens, *American Medicine*, Chapters 2, 6. See also Chapter 5, pages 75-76, of this work.

43. T. J. Hill, "Some Remarks on the Midwifery Question: Must the Midwife Perish?" *Medical Record*, 4 (October 1898), 475.

44. Abraham Jacobi, "The Best Means of Combatting Infant Mortality," *Journal of the American Medical Association*, 58 (June 1912), 1740-1744; Abraham Jacobi, "A Final Word to the Fellows and Members of the American Medical Association," *Journal of the American Medical Association*, 61 (August 1913), 635.

45. A. Elizabeth Ingraham, "History of the Bureau of Child Hygiene," *Bulletin*, Connecticut State Department of Health, 43 (April 1929), 143; *Fifty-First Annual Report*, New Jersey State Department of Health (1928), p. 154.

46. *Resolution Adopted by the Medical Association of Georgia Concerning the Practice of Midwifery in Georgia, May 9, 1924*, Georgia Department of Public Health, Miscellaneous Files, Box 1.

47. *Regulations Governing the Practice of Midwifery, January 28, 1925,* Georgia State Board of Health, Miscellaneous Files, Box 1; *Report,* Georgia State Board of Health (1931-1932), p. 32.

48. *Report,* Georgia State Board of Health (1931-1932), p. 32; Bowdoin, "The Midwife Problem," 90-92.

49. *Medical Woman's Journal,* 1 (1893) - 37 (1930). See especially the following articles, Eliza H. Root, "The Art and Science of Obstetrics," *Woman's Medical Journal,* 7 (January 1898), 24-26; Sophia Hinze Scott, "Prevention of Infant Mortality," *Woman's Medical Journal,* 21 (July 1911), 141-144; Mary Sutton Macy, "Infant Mortality, Child Hygiene and Community Life," *Woman's Medical Journal,* 26 (May 1916), 124-127; Emma Javel Neal, "Sane Obstetrics," *Medical Woman's Journal,* 30 (October 1923), 289-292. Elizabeth Jarrett, "The Midwife or the Woman Doctor," *Medical Record,* 54 (October 1898), 610-611.

The records of the American Medical Woman's Association (AMWA), founded in 1915 by a small group of militant women concerned with equal opportunity for female physicians, would most likely prove useful in determining the attitudes of women physicians toward the early twentieth-century midwife. Unfortunately, these records, which are located at the Florence A. Moore Library of Medicine, Medical College of Pennsylvania, are just now in the process of being cataloged. Moreover, the AMWA did not publish an official journal prior to 1946. Carol Lopate, *Women in Medicine* (Baltimore, 1968), p. 17; Letter from Carol Fenichel, reference librarian, Florence A. Moore Library of Medicine, Medical College of Pennsylvania, January 30, 1974.

Of course, the percentage of female physicians to male physicians was quite small during this period. In 1905, for example, 4 percent of all medical graduates were women. In 1910, however, this figure had dropped to 2.6. It did not reach the 1905 figure of 4 percent again until 1920. In 1930, women medical graduates made up 4.5 percent of all medical graduates. Lopate, *Women in Medicine,* p. 193.

50. "To Chicago's Midwives," *Topics of Interest to Midwives,* 2 (January 1918), 1.

51. For additional information on the *Progressive Midwife,* see page 96 of this chapter.

52. *Forty-Fourth Report,* Connecticut State Department of Health (1929), p. 389; "Lack of Care of American Mothers," 298.

53. *Forty-Ninth Annual Report,* New Jersey State Department of Health (1926), p. 101.

54. Statistics relating to the number of midwives who maintained full and part-time practices are scattered and incomplete. Contemporary reports indicate, however, that large numbers of women served as occasional

midwives. See, for example, *Thirty-Eighth Report*, Connecticut State Department of Health (1923), p. 253; Jessie L. Marriner, *Midwifery in Alabama* (Alabama State Board of Health [1925]), pp. 3-4, 12; Elizabeth Moore, *Maternity and Infant Care in a Rural County in Kansas*, United States Department of Labor, Children's Bureau Publication, No. 26 (Washington, D.C., 1917), pp. 22-23; Hazel Wedgewood, "Midwifery in Massachusetts," *Commonhealth*, 8 (March-April 1921), pp. 76, 78.

55. *Practice of Medicine and Midwifery in the District of Columbia.* Hearing before a subcommittee, 69th Congress, 2d session, on S. 441, to regulate the practice of medicine and midwifery in the District of Columbia and to punish persons violating provisions thereof. January 5, 1927.

56. Stevens, *American Medicine*, p. 145.

57. White House Conference on Child Health and Protection, *Obstetric Education* (New York, 1932), pp. 178-191, 195; M. Theopane Shoemaker, *History of Nurse-Midwifery in the United States* (Washington, D.C., 1947), p. 10; White House Conference on Child Health and Protection, *Public Health Organization* (New York, 1932), p. 43.

58. Sam Shapiro, Edward R. Schlesinger, and Robert E. L. Nesbitt, Jr., *Infant, Perinatal, Maternal and Childbirth Morbidity in the United States* (Cambridge, Mass., 1968), p. 4; *White House Conference on Child Health and Protection, 1930: Addresses and Abstracts of Committee Reports* (New York, 1931), p. 75; White House Conference on Child Health and Protection, *Obstetric Education*, p. 197; United States Bureau of the Census, *Vital Statistics of the United States, 1970* (Washington, D.C., 1974).

59. *White House Conference on Child Health and Protection, 1930: Addresses and Abstracts of Committee Reports*, pp. v-viii.

60. White House Conference on Child Health and Protection, *Obstetric Education*, pp. 5, 9, 198, 205, 206.

61. Ibid., pp. 216-217.

62. White House Conference on Child Health and Protection, *Fetal, Newborn, and Maternal Morbidity and Mortality* (New York, 1933), pp. 18, 217-218.

63. *Medical Care for the American People: The Final Report of the Committee on the Costs of Medical Care* (Chicago, 1932), pp. v-xi; Lloyd C. Taylor, Jr., *The Medical Profession and Social Reform, 1885-1945* (New York, 1974), pp. 122-127.

64. *Medical Care for the American People*, p. 33; Reed, *Midwives*, p. vi.

65. Reed, *Midwives*, pp. 4, 13-16, 20, 22.

66. Ransom S. Hooker, *Maternal Mortality in New York City: A Study of All Puerperal Deaths, 1930-1932* (New York, 1933), pp. x, 7.

67. Ibid., pp. 32-33, 214.

68. Ibid., pp. xi, 186, 209. See, for example, George W. Kosmak, "Certain Aspects of the Midwife Problem in Relation to the Medical Profession and Community," *Medical Record*, 85 (June 1914), 1013-1017.

69. Hooker, *Maternal Mortality*, p. 143.

70. Shapiro, Schlesinger, and Nesbitt, *Infant*, p. 145; "When Mothers Die It's News," *Nation*, 138 (January 1934), 118; "Hazards of Childbirth," *Nation*, 137 (November 1933), 612; Philadelphia County Medical Society Committee on Maternal Welfare, *Maternal Mortality in Philadelphia, 1931-1933* (Philadelphia, 1934), p. 29.

71. *Report of the Committee of the New York Obstetrical Society to Review the Maternal Mortality Report of the Public Health Relations Committee of the New York Academy of Medicine* (New York, 1934), pp. 3, 4, 7.

72. Iago Galdston, *Maternal Deaths—The Ways to Prevention* (New York, 1937), pp. 9, 50-56.

73. John Higham, *Strangers in the Land: Patterns of American Nativism, 1860-1925* (New York, 1970), p. 311; Reed, *Midwives*, p. 5; *Forty-Fourth Report*, Connecticut State Department of Health (1929), p. 387; *Forty-Ninth Annual Report*, New Jersey State Department of Health (1926), p. 100; "Midwives Dwindle Under Immigration Restrictions," *Journal of the American Medical Association*, 93 (October 1929), 1317.

74. Wilson H. Grabill, Clyde V. Kiser, and Pascal K. Whelpton, *The Fertility of American Women* (New York, 1958), pp. 3, 27; Morris Fishbein, "The Costs of High Obstetrical Care," *American Mercury*, 30 (September 1933), 62; Grace N. Fletcher, "Balancing the Baby Budget," *Century*, 89 (1925-1926), 419.

75. See, for example, M. Beatrice Blankenship, "Enduring Miracle," *Atlantic*, 152 (October 1933), 409-415; Marine Davis, "Childbirth," *Pictorial Review*, 40 (October 1938), 18-19, 66-67; Jennings C. Litzenberg, "A Child Is to Be Born," *Hygenia*, 4 (June 1926), 306-308; Louise Zabriskie, Expectant Mothers: Preparing for the Baby's Birth," *Parents' Magazine*, 6 (March 1931), 70-71.

76. United States Bureau of the Census, *Statistical Abstract of the United States: 1975* (Washington, D.C., 1975), p. 57.

7

The Rise of
Nurse-Midwifery

The concept of nurse-midwifery grew out of the midwife debate of the early years of the twentieth century. Some of the leading supporters of the trained and regulated midwife also endorsed the development of nurse-midwifery programs. For example, in 1911 Carolyn C. Van Blarcom urged "nurses in America to develop midwifery as a phase of their visiting nursing work." Similarly, Clara D. Noyes was hopeful that the midwife could "gradually be replaced by the nurse, who has, upon her general training superimposed a course in midwifery. . . ." Some midwife opponents also reluctantly supported the concept of the nurse-midwife. J. Clifton Edgar, a physician who believed that all midwives were a "necessary evil," conceded that "a graduate nurse, from a training school of good standing, can undoubtedly be trained in six months or less, to become a safe and efficient attendant upon cases of normal labor. . . ." Likewise, Dr. George W. Kosmak, who was quite critical of the practices of early twentieth-century midwives, argued in 1914 that a possible solution to this problem might be arrived at by allowing visiting nurses, "carefully trained" in prenatal and puerperal care, to attend women.[1]

The individual who was responsible for first introducing the term _nurse-midwife_ into the American vocabulary was Fred J. Taussig, a physician from St. Louis, Missouri. Taussig presented a paper to the second annual meeting of the National Organization for Public Health Nursing in 1914 in which he suggested that the solution to the "midwife question" lay in the "establishment of schools of midwifery, admission to which would be limited to graduate nurses." He was undecided as to whether such schools should maintain an independent existence or be part of the graduate department of a nurse's training school. He suggested that the curciculum include "attendance for six months to a year, entire charge of at least thirty cases of normal confinement, . . . a systematic course of lectures and demonstrations, thorough hospital training in diagnosis, [and] special work in the treatment of emergencies. . . ." Taussig also stipulated that nurse-midwifery schools should be affiliated with "hospital[s] possessing a large obstetrical material." He believed that it was more practical "to train the nurse to do midwifery than to attempt to teach the midwife some of the rudiments of nursing." Taussig concluded by stating that he thought the "nurse-midwife would prove to be the most sympathetic, the most economical, and the most efficient agent in the case of normal confinements."[2]

For the next ten years, however, few positive measures in behalf of the nurse-midwife were undertaken. A beginning step in the development of a nurse-midwifery program occurred with the establishment of New York City's Maternity Center Association (MCA) in 1918. A 1915 study of maternity care in New York City, sponsored by the city Department of Health, recommended the establishment of maternity centers throughout the city as a way to combat the high maternal and infant mortality rates. The Maternity Center Association, supported by the Women's City Club and the New York Milk Committee, was established for the purpose of setting up these centers. By 1920, thirty centers and substations had been established in nine of the ten zones in New York City. These centers helped to provide proper prenatal care for pregnant women by holding classes for expectant women, supervising patients not under other medical care, selecting the patients in need of hospital care, and aiding those women who were to be delivered in their homes.[3] With the expansion of the activities of the Maternity Center Association, its Board of Directors decided that it would be useful to employ nurses who also had training in midwifery. In 1923, an agreement was made with the Bellevue School for Midwives to allow nurses employed by the MCA to receive instructions in midwifery. The project failed, however, because the New York City commissioner of welfare refused to support it.[4]

While the work of the Maternity Center Association continued, another plan to provide pregnant women with nurse-midwifery services was underway in the mountains of Kentucky. Mary Breckinridge, a graduate nurse and native of Kentucky, began work on this project during the early 1920s. From 1919 to 1922, Breckinridge had the opportunity to observe the activities of midwives in France and England while she served with the Visiting Nurse Service of the American Committee for Devastated France. When she returned to the United States in 1922, she spent a year studying public health nursing at Columbia University. The following summer she conducted an extensive study of obstetric care in three mountain counties of Kentucky.[5]

Breckinridge spent a good part of the summer of 1923 locating the fifty-three midwives she interviewed. Most of these women lived in remote sections of the mountains where horseback was the only mode of transportation. She reported that "the midwives did not begin their practice. It was thrust upon them. As neighbors in a lonely country they were called upon for this as well as for every other emergency." Breckinridge also expressed concern over the fact that the women with whom she spoke had little training other than what their mothers or older midwives had taught them. Only twelve of the fifty-three women she interviewed could read and write. Moreover, there were very few licensed physicians upon whom the midwives could call when emergencies arose.[6]

In an attempt to try to rectify this situation, Breckinridge decided to go to England where she could receive training as a nurse-midwife. Following her certification by the Central Midwives Board, she traveled to the highlands of Scotland where she observed its nursing and maternal care program. When she returned to the United States early in 1925, she began preparations for establishing a nurse-midwifery program in the Kentucky mountains. Breckinridge believed that if a successful nurse-midwifery program could be established in the remote and poverty-stricken mountains of Kentucky that similar work could be performed anywhere in the United States.[7]

In May 1925, Breckinridge met with other concerned individuals in Frankfort, Kentucky, and formed the Kentucky Committee for Mothers and Babies. The purpose of this committee was "to safeguard the lives and health of mothers and young children by providing trained nurse-midwives for rural areas where there are no resident physicians. . . ." The sixty-three original members of the committee decided to concentrate their efforts in Leslie County, Kentucky. They immediately began work on the establishment of a nursing center in Hyden (Leslie County), Kentucky, which was staffed by American nurse-midwives who had been trained in England. Following the opening of the Hyden Center in 1925, several other nursing centers were soon established. In the meantime, Breckinridge began publishing the *Quarterly Bulletin of the Kentucky Committee for Mothers and Babies*.[8]

Over the next few years, the work of the Kentucky committee continued to expand and by 1927 it was providing maternal and child health care to women and children throughout 250 square miles of rugged Kentucky terrain. Not only did additional American nurses go to England and receive midwifery training, but midwives from England and Scotland also joined the Kentucky staff. In 1928, three years after the committee was established, the name of the organization was changed to the Frontier Nursing Service (FNS). The following year the American Association of Nurse-Midwives was created.[9]

A variety of feature stories on the Frontier Nursing Service appeared in popular periodicals during the late 1920s and early 1930s. In October 1926, *Survey* magazine awarded Mary Breckinridge a $250 cash prize for public achievement for her article, "An Adventure in Midwifery." A 1931 article, published in *American Magazine*, pointed out that only one maternal death had occurred during the 800 deliveries supervised by the FNS. *Good Housekeeping, Literary Digest*, and the *North American Review* also published articles on the Frontier Nursing Service. In addition, professional nursing journals, such as the *American Journal of Nursing* and *Public Health Nurse*, publicized the activities of the nurse-midwives of Kentucky.[10]

The success of the Frontier Nursing Service helped persuade the Committee on the Costs of Medical Care to support the development of nurse-midwifery programs. In its final report, published in 1932, the committee discussed some of the achievements of the FNS and recommended "the wider use of trained and supervised nurse-midwives as a way to improving obstetrical practice. . . ." One year later, the New York Academy of Medicine's Committee on

Public Health Relations also endorsed the concept of the nurse-midwife as well as the non-nurse-midwife.[11]

By the early 1930s, nurse-midwifery was no longer the totally unfamiliar concept it had been just twenty years earlier. Americans had had the opportunity to read about the nurse-midwife in popular magazines and nursing journals. Organizations concerned with medical reform, such as the Committee on the Costs of Medical Care and the New York Academy of Medicine, had also published information on nurse-midwifery. Moreover, the concept of the nurse-midwife was further advanced with the establishment of the Association for the Promotion and Standardization of Midwifery in 1931.[12]

The birth of this new organization was primarily the result of the work of Ralph W. Lobenstine, a New York City physician who served as chairman of the Medical Board of the Maternity Center Association from 1919-1931. He, along with several other concerned individuals including Mary Breckinridge and George W. Kosmak, founded the Association for the Promotion and Standardization of Midwifery in order to outline "the need of schools of midwifery and the principles of their control." One goal of the association was to establish a school for nurse-midwives in New York City.[13]

Shortly after the association was established, Lobenstine died. The other members of the association, however, went ahead with the plans to establish a school of nurse-midwifery. Later that year they opened the Lobenstine Midwifery Clinic and School in the center of Harlem as a memorial to Dr. Lobenstine. Only registered nurses, who had graduated from accredited schools of nursing, could enroll in the Lobenstine School. The course covered a ten-month period and included instruction in public health nursing and midwifery. Three years later, in 1934, the Lobenstine Midwifery Clinic and School was amalgamated with the Maternity Center Association under the latter's name.[14]

The work performed by the Maternity Center Association was truly commendable. Of the first 1,081 pregnant women who enrolled with the MCA , only one died. The district as a whole, however, experienced a maternal death rate of 10.4 per 1,000 live births. Graduates of the MCA also went to Alabama, Maryland, and other southern states where they assisted in the training of "grannies."

Furthermore, in 1941, the Maternity Center Association sent some of its nurse-midwives to Tuskegee, Alabama, to help set up the Tuskegee Nurse-Midwifery School. This school, which existed for six years, was established in order that black nurses from the South might be able to receive training in midwifery. Representatives from the MCA also participated in the establishment of a nurse-midwifery school in Santa Fe, New Mexico, in 1944.[15]

While the Maternity Center Association continued to expand its activities, the depression forced the Frontier Nursing Service to curtail its work. Private donations could no longer be depended upon as a source of income. One of its nursing centers was forced to close because of lack of money. England's entry into World War II in 1939 posed another serious problem to the continued existence of the FNS. Eighteen of the twenty-three nurse-midwives on the staff were British. With the outbreak of World War II, these women felt obliged to return to England. In order to insure that other nursing centers would not be shut down, the FNS immediately began to make plans for its own school. Later that year, the Frontier Graduate School of Midwifery was established.[16]

Despite the work of the Maternity Center Association and the Frontier Nursing Service, nurse-midwives have encountered numerous obstacles in their attempts to gain acceptance by the medical profession and the American public. Indeed, many of the forces responsible for the demise of the early twentieth-century lay midwife have also worked against the growth and development of nurse-midwifery programs. During the past thirty years, however, a few significant steps have been undertaken.

In 1945, for example, the "first organized attempt to develop a program of evaluation for nurse-midwifery education" occurred when the National Organization for Public Health Nursing (NOPHN) established a special section on nurse-midwifery. Throughout the 1940s and early 1950s, nurse-midwife proponents worked through the NOPHN in their attempts to set standards for nurse-midwifery education. With the reorganization of the major nursing organizations in 1952, however, the NOPHN was discontinued.[17]

The two remaining national nursing organizations, the American Nurses' Association (ANA) and the National League for Nursing (NLN) did not develop special sections on nurse-midwifery. For four years, however, nurse-midwife proponents attempted to work through the Maternal and Child Health Council of the National League for Nursing. Because this council was a medley of nursing groups including obstetrics, pediatrics, crippled children, and school nurses, it was decided that this was not the place for nurse-midwives. Following this decision, nurse-midwives in attendance at the 1954 annual convention of the ANA met together and made plans to organize a separate professional organization. As a result of this meeting, the American College of Nurse-Midwifery (ACNM) was founded in 1955. In 1969, the American College of Nurse-Midwifery joined with the Kentucky-based American Association of Nurse-Midwives and formed the American College of Nurse-Midwives.[18]

From its inception in 1955, the American College of Nurse-Midwives has been concerned with "the need for objective evaluation and rating of educational programs in nurse-midwifery. . . ." Editorials published in its official bulletin have insisted that the ACNM is the logical group to establish accreditation programs. At the present time, the American College of Nurse-Midwives publishes a list of approved nurse-midwifery programs. Graduates of these programs are then eligible to take the ACNM national examination for certification.[19]

Another concern of the American College of Nurse-Midwives has been the question of the legal recognition of the nurse-midwife. In 1945, New Mexico formally recognized the nurse-midwife. No other area of the country enacted similar legislation until 1959 when New York City provided for her licensing. Due primarily to the lobbying efforts of the ACNM, additional states began to enact regulatory legislation during the 1960s and early 1970s. As of May 1975, no state clearly prohibited the practice of nurse-midwifery. In five states, however, nurse-midwives were not permitted to practice fully due to restrictive interpretations of the laws. In seventeen additional states, moreover, nurse-midwives were not practicing fully, even though there were no state laws preventing them from doing so.[20]

Maternal and infant mortality rates across the United States have experienced sharp reductions in those areas where nurse-midwives have been fully utilized. For example, the Frontier Nursing Service experienced only eleven maternal deaths during its first 10,000 deliveries between 1925 and 1954. In contrast, the national maternal mortality rate per 10,000 live births for the years 1939-1941 was 36.3. The low maternal death rate of the FNS was especially significant since "60 percent of deliveries between 1925 and 1954 were conducted in the home in an extremely poverty-stricken area, where the main mode of transportation was by horseback, modern facilities and medical assistance were difficult to attain, and the percentage of high-risk mothers and infants was great." Since 1952, moreover, there have been no maternal deaths in over 8,000 deliveries, and the stillbirth and neonatal mortality rates of the FNS continue to decline.[21] Similarly, Madera County, California, and target areas in Mississippi have experienced sharp reductions in their infant mortality rates with the introduction of nurse-midwifery programs.[22]

Although the utilization of nurse-midwives has resulted in improved health care for mothers and babies, the medical profession and the public have been reluctant to endorse the concept of nurse-midwifery. Frequently, the nurse-midwife of the present is confused with the lay midwife of the early twentieth century. Moreover, the term *midwife* often invokes negative connotations. In fact, one recently published article suggests that part of the slow acceptance of the nurse-midwife "is due to the fact that the crusaders who set out to eradicate unskilled midwifery early in the century did their job perhaps too well."[23]

Modern-day critics of the nurse-midwife, such as Dr. Russell J. Paalman, often echo the arguments voiced by many of the early twentieth-century midwife opponents. Paalman, in his presidential address to the forty-second annual meeting of the Central Association of Obstetricians and Gynecologists, expressed dismay over the fact that "many highly respected obstetricians" had supported the nurse-midwife "as a stopgap for the alleged doctor shortage." He argued that "if modern obstetrics, available in most places in our country, were available everywhere and the birth rate continues below 2.0, why do we need them?" In language characteristic of the early twentieth-century midwife opponents, Paalman stated:

Can a nurse-midwife pick up all the early signs of impending disaster and consult an obstetrician in time? Is not every pregnant woman entitled to a trained obstetrician's care and delivery in a modern obstetric suite? By 1980, there should be an oversupply of obstetricians. Except in a very few deprived areas, is there a place for nurse-midwives in the United States? I think not![24]

Not all physicians, however, have taken such a negative approach to the concept of nurse-midwifery. For example, the American Medical Association, while not adopting a formal policy statement on nurse-midwifery, has expressed "tacit approval" of all organizations which represent the nurse-midwife. Some doctors, moreover, are openly optimistic about the nurse-midwife's role within the American medical system. Writing for *Obstetrics and Gynecology* in February 1971, Dr. John Van S. Maeck stated that the midwife "has an extremely important role to play in newly developing sytems of maternal and child health care. Because of her training, she is qualified to manage the uncomplicated pregnancy and labor and to recognize the abnormal." Furthermore, Maeck argued that the proper utilization of nurse-midwives would enable obstetricians to devote more of their time to high-risk patients.[25]

One of the most significant pronouncements in behalf of nurse-midwifery was issued early in 1971, when the American College of Obstetricians and Gynecologists adopted a formal policy statement which recognized that "the deficits in availability and quality of maternity care can best be corrected by the cooperative efforts of teams of physicians, nurse-midwives, obstetric registered nurses and other health personnel." The statement specified that "in such medically directed teams, qualified nurse-midwives may assume responsibility for the complete care and management of uncomplicated maternity patients."[26] Nevertheless, the percentage of births attended by nurse-midwives remains quite small. As late as 1973, in fact, less than 1 percent of all births in the United States were attended by both nurse-midwives *and* non-nurse-midwives.[27]

It is interesting to note how the concept of nurse-midwifery has evolved since Dr. Fred J. Taussig first introduced the term into the American vocabulary in 1914. Taussig, like other early nurse-midwife proponents, was insistent that the nurse-midwife be a graduate nurse who had received special training in midwifery. When the American College of Nurse-Midwives formulated its official position on the nurse-midwife, it specified that she be a registered nurse who by virtue of her added knowledge and skill gained through an organized program of study and clinical experience recognized by the American College of Nurse-Midwifery, has extended the limits . . . of her practice into the area of management of cases of mothers and babies throughout the maternity cycle so long as progress meets criteria accepted as normal.

Similarly, the American Nurses' Association's first formal statement on nurse-midwifery, issued in 1968, emphasized that the nurse-midwife was, first of all, a professional nurse. In the same year, the ACNM reemphasized that nurse-midwifery was "a clinical specialty in nursing."[28]

During the early 1970s, however, a movement was initiated to have nurse-midwifery recognized as a profession in itself. Several articles to this effect were published in the *Journal of Nurse-Midwifery,* the official publication of the ACNM. For example, Mary Swelting, a certified nurse-midwife, called for enabling legislation which would separate nurse-midwifery from medicine and nursing "for the midwife is neither a nurse practitioner nor a junior medical practitioner." She believed that "calling ourselves midwives . . . will increase the public's awareness of our true professional identity and facilitate the return of the honorable profession of midwifery to the United States." Another article argued that "in resurrecting the midwife, it was necessary to create the midwife from the nursing discipline which was held in the highest esteem. . . . [but] as with every birthing process, it is time now to cut the umbilical cord." At the present time, however, nurse-midwifery is officially defined as a specialty within nursing.[29]

Despite the reluctance of the medical profession and the public to accept the nurse-midwife, the American College of Nurse-Midwives is quite optimistic about her future. In 1971, the ACNM reported that it had located 1,256 nurse-midwives in the United States. Two years later, it published a list of seventeen approved educational programs in nurse-midwifery, including the courses offered by the Frontier Nursing Service and the Maternity Center Association. Moreover, between 1968 and 1971 the United States experienced a 14 percent increase of "nurse-midwives employed in direct nurse-midwifery service." Thus, it is not surprising that a 1972 study conducted by the ACNM concluded that "the American nurse-midwife is part of a dynamic growing group making a significant contribution . . . in the provision of comprehensive maternity care."[30]

NOTES

1. Carolyn C. Van Blarcom, "Visiting Obstetrical Nursing," *Transactions of the American Association for the Study and Prevention of Infant Mortality*, 2 (1911), 349; Clara D. Noyes, "The Training of Midwives in Relation to the Prevention of Infant Mortality," *American Journal of Obstetrics and the Diseases of Women and Children*, 66 (1912), 1057; J. Clifton Edgar, "The Education, Licensing and Supervision of the Midwife," *American Journal of Obstetrics and the Diseases of Women and Children*, 73 (March 1916), 391; George W. Kosmak, "Certain Aspects of the Midwife Problem in Relation to the Medical Profession and the Community," *Medical Record*, 85 (June 1914), 1015.

2. Fred J. Taussig, "The Nurse-Midwife," *Public Health Nurse Quarterly*, 6 (October 1914), 33-35, 39.

3. *Forty-Fifth Annual Report and Log, 1915-1963, of the Maternity Center Association* [1964], pp. 1-3.

4. M. Theopane Shoemaker, *History of Nurse-Midwifery in the United States* (Washington, D.C., 1947), p. 12.

5. Mary Breckinridge, *Wide Neighborhoods: A Story of the Frontier Nursing Service* (New York, 1952), pp. 111-116.

6. Mary Breckinridge, "Midwifery in the Kentucky Mountains, An Investigation in 1923," *Quarterly Bulletin of the Frontier Nursing Service*, 17 (Spring 1942), 34, 38, 40.

7. Breckinridge, *Wide Neighborhoods*, pp. 124-127, 158.

8. Ibid., pp. 159-161; Shoemaker, *History of Nurse-Midwifery*, pp. 17-19.

9. Shoemaker, *History of Nurse-Midwifery* pp. 20-21; Breckinridge, *Wide Neighborhoods*, p. 305.

10. Mary Breckinridge, "An Adventure in Midwifery," *Survey*, 57 (October 1926), 25-27, 47; H. Worden, "She Nurses Her Patients for a Dollar a Year," *American Magazine*, 112 (December 1931), 69-70; E. Poole, "Nurse on Horseback: Frontier Nursing Service," *Good Housekeeping*, 94 (June 1932), 38-39, 203-210; Edith R. Solenberger, "Nurses on Horseback, Frontier Nursing Service," *Hygenia*, 9 (July 1931), 633-638; Mary Breckinridge, "Hard-Riding Nurses of Kentucky," *Literary Digest*, 96 (March 1928), 29-30; Mary Breckinridge, "Maternity in the Mountains," *North American Review*, 226 (December 1928), 765-768; "Midwifery in Kentucky," *American Journal of Nursing*, 25 (December 1925), 1004; E. C. Rockstroh, "Enter the Nurse-Midwife," *American Journal of Nursing*, 27 (March 1927), 159-164; "The Frontier Nursing Service," *American Journal of Nursing*,

31 (January 1931), 44; Alice Logan, "The Nurse-Midwife in Leslie County, Kentucky," *Public Health Nurse*, 18 (1926), 542-546.

11. *Medical Care for the American People: The Final Report of the Committee on the Costs of Medical Care* (Chicago, 1932), pp. 33, 112, 143; Ransom S. Hooker, *Maternal Mortality in New York City: A Study of All Puerperal Deaths, 1930-1932* (New York, 1933), p. 210.

12. "A Training School for Nurse-Midwives Established," *American Journal of Nursing*, 32 (April 1932), 374.

13. Ibid.; *Forty-Fifth Annual Report and Log, 1915-1963, of the Maternity Center Association* [1964], pp. 8-9; Shoemaker, *History of Nurse-Midwifery*, pp. 8-9.

14. "A Training School for Nurse-Midwives Established," 374; Maternity Center Association, *Twenty Years of Nurse-Midwifery, 1933-1953* (New York, [1955]), pp. 17-18.

15. Maternity Center Association, *Twenty Years*, pp. 39, 54-61.

16. Shoemaker, *History of Nurse-Midwifery*, p. 23; Dorothy F. Buck, "The Nurses on Horseback Ride On," *American Journal of Nursing*, 40 (March 1940), 993-995; "Courses for Nurse-Midwives," *American Journal of Nursing*, 40 (March 1940), 335.

17. *Education for Nurse-Midwifery: The Report of the Work Conference on Nurse-Midwifery* (New York, 1958), p. 46; Letter from Aileen Hogan, chairwoman, Archives Committee, American College of Nurse-Midwives, July 11, 1974.

18. Letter from Aileen Hogan, July 11, 1974; *Nurse-Midwife Bulletin*, 1 (May 1954; July 1954); "Editorial," *Bulletin of the American College of Nurse-Midwives*, 14 (August 1969), 68.

19. Cecelia Sehl, "Accreditation in Higher Education," *Bulletin of the American College of Nurse-Midwifery*, 5 (June 1960), 36-38; Vera Keane, "Accreditation and Responsibility," *Bulletin of the American College of Nurse-Midwifery*, 5 (June 1960), 39-41; *What Is a Nurse-Midwife?* (New York, 1973); Letter from Aileen Hogan, July 11, 1974.

20. David Harris, "The Development of Nurse-Midwifery in New York City," *Bulletin of the American College of Nurse-Midwifery*, 14 (February 1969), 9; "Patterns of Legislation and Actual Practice of Nurse-Midwifery in States and Jurisdictions," *Journal of Nurse-Midwifery*, 21 (Summer 1976), 13. The authors of a recent survey of nurse-midwifery legislation throughout the United States suggest that "conservative attitudes of doctors, hospital administrators, and nursing leaders, or restrictive third-party payment policies of health insurance companies, or unsuitable salaries and working conditions" may be "significant factors that prevent full practice by nurse-midwives." "Conclusions," *Journal of Nurse-Midwifery*, 21 (Summer 1976), 19.

21. Helen E. Browne and Gertrude Isaacs, "The Frontier Nursing Service: The Primary Care Nurse in the Community Hospital," *American Journal of Obstetrics and Gynecology,* 124 (January 1976), 16.

22. Barry S. Levy, Frederick S. Wilkinson, and William M. Marine, "Reducing Neonatal Mortality Rate with Nurse-Midwives," *American Journal of Obstetrics and Gynecology,* 109 (January 1971), 50-58; Marie C. Meglen and Helen V. Burst, "Nurse-Midwives Make a Difference," *Nursing Outlook,* 22 (June 1974), 386-389.

23. Phyllis Burosh, "Physicians' Attitudes Toward Nurse-Midwives," *Nursing Outlook,* 23 (July 1975)', 453-456; Seth B. Goldsmith, John W.C. Johnson, and Monroe Lerner, "Obstetricians' Attitudes Toward Nurse-Midwives," *American Journal of Obstetrics and Gynecology,* 111 (September 1971), 111-118; John Van S. Maeck, "Obstetrician-Midwife Partnership in Obstetric Care," *Obstetrics and Gynecology,* 37 (February 1971), 316; Macy Foundation, *The Training and Responsibilities of the Midwife* (New York, 1967), p. 154; "Rebirth of the Midwife," *Life,* 71 (November 1971), 50-55; Dorothy Crane Davis and Lamar Middleton, "Rebirth of the Midwife," *Today's Health* (February 1968), 28-31, 70-71.

24. Russell J. Paalman, "The Abundant Life: Presidential Address," *American Journal of Obstetrics and Gynecology,* 122 (May 1975), 140.

25. Letter from Naomi Patchin, director of the Section on Nursing, American Medical Association, August 12, 1975; Maeck, "Obstetrician-Midwife Partnership," 317.

26. "Joint Statement on Maternity Care," *Journal of Nurse-Midwifery,* 20 (Fall 1975), 15.

27. United States Bureau of the Census, *Statistical Abstract of the United States: 1975* (Washington, D.C., 1975), p. 57.

28. Taussig, "The Nurse-Midwife," 34-35; "Statement of Functions, Standards and Qualification for Practice of Nurse-Midwives," *Bulletin of the American College of Nurse-Midwifery,* 9 (Winter 1964), 80; "ANA Statement on Nurse-Midwifery," *Bulletin of the American College of Nurse-Midwifery,* 13 (February 1968), 26-27; *Education for Nurse-Midwifery: The Report of the Second Work Conference on Nurse-Midwifery Education* (New York, 1967), p. 45.

29. Mary Swelting, "Letters to the Editor," *Journal of Nurse-Midwifery,* 18 (Spring 1973), 3; "Editorial," *Journal of Nurse-Midwifery,* 18 (Fall 1973), 3. See also Lucille Woodville, "Letters to the Editor," *Journal of Nurse-Midwifery,* 19 (Spring 1974), 4-5; Letter from Aileen Hogan, July 11, 1974.

30. Research Committee of the American College of Nurse-Midwives, *Descriptive Data: Nurse-Midwives—U.S.A.* (New York, [1972]), pp. 2, 6, 14; *What Is a Nurse-Midwife?*; Ruth M. White, "A Nurse-Midwife Looks Ahead," *Journal of Nurse-Midwifery,* 19 (Fall 1974), 4-10.

8

Conclusion

Most births in the United States were attended by midwives prior to 1910. Early in American history, however, male physicians began to make inroads into the lying-in chamber. In the 1760s, for example, William Shippen, Jr., a physician from Philadelphia, began offering instruction in midwifery for women as well as for men. Advances in obstetric knowledge, especially the development of the forceps, and the establishment of all-male medical schools further enabled physicians to gain acceptance as accoucheurs. By 1800, in fact, it was quite fashionable for upper-class American women in urban areas to enlist physicians as accoucheurs for ordinary labors.

As the nineteenth century progressed, the number of male midwives continued to grow. Nevertheless, the desire to maintain decency and morality in the lying-in chamber prevented many Americans from accepting physicians as birth attendants for normal deliveries. The advancement of medical professionalism and new discoveries in the field of obstetrics enabled physicians to convince many middle- and upper-class Americans that the well-being and safety of the parturient woman were more important than preserving decency in the lying-in chamber. By the decade of the 1860s, in fact, male physicians no longer found it necessary to battle for the right to enter the lying-in chamber. They had won acceptance as accoucheurs among urban, middle- and upper-class Americans.

During the second half of the nineteenth century, it appeared that the midwife was quietly fading from the American setting. Most late nineteenth-century manuals for pregnant women and mothers were written with the assumption that the parturient woman would hire a physician and monthly nurse for confinement. Moreover, the middle and upper classes were beginning to embrace the view that childbirth was a complicated and dangerous procedure which could most properly be controlled by the use of instruments, drugs, and surgery. The growth of medical professionalism and new obstetric discoveries seemed to insure that American midwives would eventually be displaced by physicians. Consequently, most late nineteenth-century medical practitioners, as well as most middle- and upper-class Americans, complacently ignored the midwife. Nevertheless, midwives continued to attend at least as many births as did physicians throughout the nineteenth century. As late as 1910, in fact, the commissioner of health of New York City conservatively estimated that 50 percent of all births in the United States were attended by midwives.

Although the turn-of-the-century midwife was numerically significant, middle- and upper-class Americans had little firsthand contact with her. They usually relied on the services of the general practitioner and monthly nurse. Moreover, a growing number of well-to-do women were even choosing to have their babies in hospitals where they could be attended by obstetric specialists.

In contrast, immigrants, blacks, and other poor people almost always employed the midwife. They could not afford to pay the high fees of physicians, and they were opposed to entering lying-in charities where they were allegedly subjected to obstetric interference and experimentation. In addition, many immigrants and blacks were opposed to having men serve as birth attendants. Finally, poor people preferred the midwife, or "granny" as she was affectionately called, because she engaged in a variety of housewifely duties not performed by the doctor.

Very few satisfactory training programs for midwives existed at the turn of the twentieth century. Most women received their training from older midwives or from physicians who awarded certificates in midwifery to virtually anyone who could afford to pay the $150 "tuition" fee. Occasionally, physicians attempted to establish quality schools for midwives. The College of Midwifery of New York City (1883), the Playfair School of Midwifery in Chicago, Illinois (1896), and the St. Louis, Missouri College of Midwifery (1895) were three such schools. For the most part, however, the educational and training programs made available to midwives at this time were highly inadequate.

During the first two decades of the twentieth century two major developments occurred which caused the medical profession, public health officials, and lay people to take note of the midwife. First, physicians became increasingly concerned about medical education reform and the related issue of "overcrowding" in the profession. Doctors maintained that overcrowding had resulted in a loss of their status and a diminution of their income. Many physicians believed that eliminating the midwife, or at least substantially reducing her numbers, would help alleviate this problem. The second, and equally significant, development was the revelation that the maternal and infant mortality rates in the United States were alarmingly high. For example, the 1910 infant mortality rate of the United States was 124 deaths per 1,000 live births. Moreover, the federal Children's Bureau reported in 1917 that "childbirth caused more deaths among women fifteen to forty-four years old than any disease except tuberculosis."[1] The bureau also reported that only two of fifteen countries it had investigated had maternal mortality rates higher than the United States for the 1900-1910 period. The infant mortality rate of the United States was also substantially higher than that reported by some of the major countries of Europe. Once these birth and death statistics were made public, physicians and health officials began to question the midwife's role in the birth process and to try to determine why so many American mothers and infants were dying.

By 1910, physicians, and to a lesser extent the general public, were embroiled in a fierce debate over the present and future role of the midwife. The "midwife problem" was frequently discussed at the meetings of the various medical societies. Numerous articles on this topic appeared in medical journals throughout the United States. Popular magazines also carried feature stories on the midwife. At the same time, states began to enact new laws or to revise already existing laws pertaining to midwives. New York City led the way in midwife training and control with the establishment of the municipally sponsored Bellevue School for Midwives in 1911. In addition, the United States Children's Bureau, founded in 1912 as a division within the United States Department of Labor, helped states throughout the nation to establish midwife programs. By 1924, every state in the union had established a bureau of child hygiene or its equivalent. One of the concerns of these bureaus was how to deal with the midwife problem.

The height of the midwife debate occurred between 1910 and 1920. Physicians, many of whom were obstetric specialists, engineered the anti-midwife campaign. They believed that the obstetrician would never receive due recognition as long as women, untrained in the medical sciences, continued to attend one-half of all births. They also argued that childbirth was a potentially dangerous and complicated condition requiring the services of a highly trained physician. Thus, they were often critical of the work of general practitioners, as well as that of midwives. The American Association for the Study and Prevention of Infant Mortality (AASPIM), founded in 1910, served as a sounding board for midwife opponents. Numerous papers on the midwife problem and the degraded status of obstetrics were presented to its annual meetings.

Part of the opposition to the midwife was a result of the anti-immigrant and anti-black prejudices of the period. Opponents often issued statements to this effect. Interestingly, however, anti-midwife physicians did not find it necessary to employ the often-repeated allegation that women were biologically and intellectually inferior to men. The distinctions between the midwife and the physician were clearly delineated by the early years of the twentieth century. A woman did not have to be a man's equal in order to become a midwife. The question at issue was not whether women were qualified to be midwives, but whether anyone, other than a highly trained medical practitioner, was capable of competently practicing obstetrics.

Most of the support for the midwife originated from public health officials who believed that the maternal and infant mortality rates would be substantially reduced if midwives were properly trained and regulated. They pointed out that the maternal and infant mortality rates of many European countries were well below those of the United States, even though the percentage of midwife-attended births was much higher. The country with which the United States was most often compared was England, whose infant and maternal death rates had been significantly reduced with the passage of the 1902 Midwives Act. Proponents also publicized the fact that those localities in the United States, such as New York City and New Jersey, which had established comprehensive training programs for midwives had also experienced a reduction in their infant and maternal mortality rates.

It was not always easy to distinguish the midwife opponents from the proponents. For example, many midwife critics supported training and regulatory programs as temporary measures to be discontinued as soon as adequate numbers of physicians were properly trained. Health officials in several states, including Alabama, Mississippi, Pennsylvania, and Virginia, worked diligently to establish comprehensive programs for midwives. The ultimate goal of these officials, however, was to regulate the midwife out of existence. By contrast, similar programs were adopted in states, such as Connecticut and New Jersey, where health officials did *not* favor the ultimate elimination of the midwife. Thus, while the state bureaus of child hygiene often adopted similar training and regulatory programs, the health officials who administered these programs frequently held differing opinions as to whether or not the midwife deserved a permanent place in American society. In addition, some anti-midwife physicians were optimistic that nurses, who had received special training in obstetrics, could be substituted for midwives.

By the 1920s much of the furor of the midwife debate had tapered off. The major reason for this change of focus was that fewer and fewer births were being attended by midwives. Reports from throughout the United States indicated that the ranks of midwives were sharply and steadily decreasing. By 1930, in fact, only 15 percent of all births were attended by midwives.

A variety of factors contributed to the decline of the midwife. Certainly, the physician's argument that obstetrics was a complicated medical specialty that demanded the services of a bona fide medical practitioner played a major role in bringing about her demise. Many people were impressed with the physician's argument that maternal and infant death rates would not be substantially reduced until childbirth was recognized to be a complicated medical condition. The increased incidence of forceps deliveries and cesarean sections, as well as the development of Twilight Sleep, served to bolster this position. Furthermore, many physicians stipulated that these new childbirth techniques were to be performed in hospitals. A few doctors even argued that, ideally, all births should occur in hospitals.

Second, midwife opponents were better organized and more articulate than midwife proponents. Physicians who felt that the status of obstetrics needed to be upgraded sounded forth loudly against the midwife. They published articles in medical journals and popular magazines, read papers at the annual meetings of various medical societies, and were active members of the American Association for the Study and Prevention of Infant Mortality. What began around 1910 as an internal debate within the medical profession over the degraded status of the obstetrician resulted twenty years later in a full-fledged campaign to convince the public that childbirth was a dangerous procedure requiring the services of a specially trained physician.

By contrast, poverty, language barriers, and geographical separation helped to insure that midwives would remain isolated from each other. They had no medium, such as the American Association for the Study and Prevention of Infant Mortality, through which they could make their voices heard. Some state bureaus of child hygiene helped midwives form educational clubs and associations. These organizations, however, wielded very little political or professional power. In addition, only two journals were published expressly for American midwives during the 1900-1930 period. Both of these journals, *Topics of Interest to Midwives,* published in Chicago in 1918, and the *Progressive Midwife,* a publication of the New Jersey Bureau of Child Hygiene which first appeared in 1927, reached only a very small segment of the total number of American midwives. Thus, midwives had to depend on public health nurses, health officials, sympathetic physicians, and other concerned individuals to speak out for them. At a time when "medicine was becoming an institutionalized, collective occupation," midwives were forced to go their separate ways.[2]

A third reason for the rapid decline of the midwife was that the money appropriated for training and regulatory programs was pitifully small. Even model programs, such as those developed in New York City, New Jersey, and Connecticut, suffered from a lack of funds. The passage by the United States Congress of the Sheppard-Towner Maternity and Infancy Protection Act of 1921 provided additional funds for midwife training and regulation. Unfortunately, even these funds were quite meager. The act allotted an annual appropriation of $1,240,000 for the development of maternal and child health programs. This money was distributed to the various states on a population percentage and matching basis. Only part of this appropriation was used for developing midwife programs. Moreover, when the act was allowed to expire in 1929, many states were forced to curtail their midwife activities.

Fourth, the medley of regulatory legislation that was enacted between 1900 and 1930 also contributed to the midwife's downfall. Massachusetts was the only state to outlaw the midwife. Other states, however, were hopeful that she would eventually be regulated out of existence. Even states, such as Connecticut and New Jersey, which were sympathetic to the midwife's plight, noted that their strict supervisory programs had resulted in a reduction of her numbers.

For the most part, however, the laws pertaining to midwives were quite lenient. They usually required that she register all births and apply silver nitrate to the newborn infant's eyes as an ophthalmia prophylaxis. The laws often prohibited her from administering drugs and using instruments, performing vaginal examinations, and attending abnormal births. Some states, moreover, enacted no midwife legislation. The 1930 White House Conference on Child Health and Protection reported that ten states neither licensed nor controlled their midwives. Six other states required their midwives to be registered, but not licensed. Several states provided no penalties for violating the law, and in many areas the laws were unenforceable.

Social and cultural changes, only peripherally related to the early twentieth-century midwife debate, also helped to bring about the midwife's demise. Significantly, these changes tended to support the position of the anti-midwife physicians. For example, the rapid growth of American hospitals after 1910 freed additional beds for maternity cases. In addition, the development of the automobile provided pregnant women with a relatively quick and easy mode of transportation to the hospital. The immigration restriction laws of the early 1920s resulted in fewer women demanding the services of the midwife. By 1930, in fact, 80 percent of all midwives were reported to be living in the South. Moreover, the United States experienced its "first sustained decline in the absolute number of annual births . . . between 1921 and 1933."[3] This decline in the birth rate caused more and more people to perceive the birth of babies as very special events which required the skills of a highly trained physician.

In the midst of the early twentieth-century midwife debate, a few physicians and public health advocates began to endorse the concept of the trained and regulated nurse-midwife as a possible solution to the midwife problem. Unlike the old-style midwife who usually had no background in nursing, the nurse-midwife was a qualified nurse who also had special training in obstetrics. During the 1920s and 1930s, the Maternity Center Association of New York City and the Frontier Nursing Service, a Kentucky-based organization, paved the way for the establishment of the first schools of nurse-midwifery in the United States. In 1931 the Lobenstine Midwifery Clinic and School was established in New York City. Eight years later, the Frontier Graduate School of Midwifery was founded in Hyden, Kentucky. During the 1930s, some of the state bureaus of child hygiene began to employ graduates of these two schools to teach short courses in obstetrics to immigrant and black midwives.

The number of women trained as nurse-midwives in the 1930s was quite small. As time progressed, additional programs were gradually created. The expansion of nurse-midwifery activities throughout the United States resulted in the formulation of the American College of Nurse-Midwives (ACNM) in 1955. Since its inception, the ACNM has been primarily concerned with evaluating and rating the educational programs in nurse-midwifery and in attaining legal recognition for the nurse-midwife. Nevertheless, the concept of the nurse-midwife has won acceptance only slowly. The public frequently confuses the nurse-midwife of the present with the lay midwife of the early twentieth century. As late as 1973, in fact, less than 1 percent of all births in the United States were attended by nurse-midwives and non-nurse-midwives. Significantly, the status of the nurse-midwife appears to have improved in recent years. Between 1968 and 1971, for example, the United States experienced a 14 percent increase of "nurse-midwives employed in direct nurse-midwifery service."[4] Moreover, early in 1971, the American College of Obstetricians and Gynecologists adopted a formal policy statement in support of the nurse-midwife as part of the obsteric team. For the most part, however, the forces responsible for the demise of the early twentieth-century lay midwife have also worked against the growth and development of nurse-midwifery programs.

During the decade of the 1970s, a variety of organizations and individuals concerned with providing family-centered maternity care and restoring home childbirth in the United States began working for the revival of lay midwifery. Organizations, such as the Association for Childbirth at Home (ACAH), Home Oriented Maternity Experience (HOME), Homebirth Inc., and the National Association of Parents and Professionals for Safe Alternatives in Childbirth (NAPSAC), have become increasingly critical of the impersonal, mechanized approach to childbirth adopted by many American hospitals. In addition, women's liberation proponents, most notably the Boston Women's Health Collective, have begun to question conventional hospital birth practices and to criticize the treatment that pregnant women receive from obstetricians and other hospital personnel. These critics question the value of hospital obstetric procedures such as the shaving of pubic hair, fetal monitoring, chemical stimulation of labor, routine episiotomies, and the separation of the mother from her newborn infant. They feel that sophisticated equipment and obstetric techniques have transformed a natural and joyous event into an unnatural and much feared ordeal.[5] Many critics of hospital births believe that parturition will not be restored to its "natural state" until childbirth at home becomes a reasonable and safe alternative for healthy women throughout the United States. Moreover, they feel that the revival and legal recognition of lay midwifery will help to ensure that safe home childbirth programs are established.[6]

While home childbirth proponents welcome the support of physicians and nurse-midwives, they also maintain that individuals trained to deliver babies in hospitals do not necessarily make the best home birth attendants.[7] For example, Lester Dessez Hazell, a leading spokeswoman for the home birth movement, argues that

extensive experience in the hospital doesn't prepare a doctor or nurse to do home deliveries. . . . [W]hat is normal in the hospital may not be normal at home and vice versa. . . . In general, lay people who acknowledge their limitations are far less likely to cause problems than doctors, nurses, and others who . . . try to force what is happening in the mold of what they know. . . .[8]

Similarly, Suzanne Arms, in her book, *Immaculate Deception: A New Look at Women and Childbirth in America*, specifically explains why she feels that American nurse-midwives are often unqualified to attend home births. Arms contrasts the lay midwife who "takes great personal pride in her ability to keep nature on its course and her direct involvement with a laboring woman and her family" with the nurse-midwife who "is taught to expect anything and everything to go awry during birth, and . . . [who] has a lusty respect for modern forms of interference which will protect woman from her own working body." Arms also believes that "it is a rare nurse who leaves her training unscarred by that emphasis and expectation of disease or disorder. Thus . . . the *nurse* takes her place on the growing obstetric team, but the *midwife* has changed and lost her essence in the process." Other modern-day proponents of lay midwifery point out that the shortage of nurse-midwifery training programs in the United States, coupled with the reluctance of nurse-midwives to attend home births, necessitates the utilization of lay midwives.[9]

The American College of Nurse-Midwives is keenly aware of the growing home birth movement in the United States. In fact, the Executive Board of the ACNM adopted a position statement on home birth in October 1973, endorsing the "hospital or officially approved maternity home as the site for childbirth. . . ."[10] Not all nurse-midwives, however, agree with this position. For example, a letter from six nurse-midwives from northern California was published in the Spring 1975 issue of the *Journal of Nurse-Midwifery* urging the ACNM to reconsider its position on home birth "in the interest of professional growth in a constantly changing health care system." Likewise, an article by Charlotte Theriault Houde described the growing concern which she and other nurse-midwives were experiencing because of the "increasing number of requests for home deliveries" which they could not honor. Houde stated that she knew that there was "an underground of lay midwives in the

Northeast who . . . [were] attempting to meet the demands of consumers." She then posed the following unanswered questions: "How long can we continue to remain ostrich like? What are our ethical responsibilities in this regard?"[11]

The legal status of the contemporary lay midwife varies from state to state. A study of lay midwifery licensing requirements conducted by the Center of Law and Social Policy for HOME reported that as of July 1976 lay midwives could legally practice in twenty-four states. In five of these states, however, lay midwifery licenses are no longer issued, although midwives who were licensed in the past are permitted to continue their practice.[12]

It is difficult to determine just how many lay midwives presently attend births in the United States. One recent study suggests that nearly 5,000 "grannies" live in the rural areas of the South.[13] In addition, there are an untold number of younger lay midwives who are involved in the home birth movement. These younger women, who have often had home births themselves, frequently begin their practice by helping out friends and neighbors who also desire home childbirth. They usually read a variety of technical books on midwifery and serve apprenticeships with other midwives before actually taking on the full responsibilities of the midwife. Moreover, they usually arrange back-up services with local physicians to ensure that unforeseen emergencies are treated promptly and properly.[14]

When possible, these younger women qualify to practice under state lay midwifery laws. In Texas, for example, lay midwives must merely register with local health officials in order to practice legally. One Texas lay midwife, Shari Daniels, a former schoolteacher with a master's degree in guidance and counseling, has even established a Maternity Center in El Paso, Texas, where she conducts childbirth education classes, attends births, and trains prospective lay midwives. Daniels's training program, which consists of one or two years of study, includes instruction in prenatal care, nutrition, childbirth preparation, and midwifery practice and skills. In addition, Daniels expects her pupils to attend approximately forty births before beginning their own midwifery practice.[15]

In other areas of the United States, however, lay midwives have encountered serious legal problems in their efforts to qualify under state midwifery laws. Fran Ventre, a practicing lay midwife who is presently working toward a degree in nurse-midwifery, was forced to resort to the threat of legal action in order to obtain a lay mid-wifery license from Maryland.[16] Moreover, in many localities, lay midwives practice outside the domain of the law. In 1974, for example, three lay midwives from the Santa Cruz, California, Birth Center were arrested for practicing medicine without a license. Despite these arrests, many California midwives continue to attend home births.[17]

The strength of the lay midwifery movement was demonstrated in January 1977 when approximately 200 lay midwives from through-out the United States traveled to El Paso, Texas, to attend the First International Conference of Practicing Midwives. The conference, which was organized by three prominent lay midwives, Shari Daniels, Nancy Mills, and Fran Ventre, was called for the purpose of bringing "midwives together to share and learn." Many of the leading lay midwife proponents in the United States participated in the conference, including Raven Lang, author of *Birth Book* and founder of the Santa Cruz, California, Birth Center, Ina May, head midwife for The Farm, a spiritual community in Summertown, Tennessee, and Nancy Mills, a practicing midwife for the past seven years who has been responsible for over 450 births in Sonoma County, California. During the conference, plans were made for the establishment of regional midwifery associations and news-letters. Moreover, there was a great deal of discussion concerning the desirability of formulating competency standards for midwives and developing a national program to encourage favorable mid-wifery legislation.[18] Unlike the "grannies" of the early twentieth century, modern-day lay midwives have joined together to establish newsletters, formulate midwifery competency standards, and lobby for midwifery legislation.[19]

Significantly, the available, but limited, statistics relating to infant and maternal deaths associated with home births attended by contemporary lay midwives in the United States indicate that these figures are quite low. For example, a recent study based on a series of 287 home births assisted by midwives from the Santa Cruz, California, Birth Center, conducted by Dr. Lewis E. Mehl and Gail H. Peterson, revealed that "84% of the home deliveries were entirely normal." Of the 287 women who began labor at home, 45 "required intervention at a hospital to complete their labor." There was one stillbirth and there were no maternal deaths. The authors of this study suggested that a variety of factors probably contributed to the "good results obtained by the Birth Center women," including the screening out of high-risk patients, the avoidance of pain-relieving medication, the position the women assumed during parturition, and the lack of fear experienced by pregnant women in the presence of loving friends and familiar surroundings. Mehl and Peterson concluded that "home delivery, then, would seem to be a safe reality . . . especially . . . when the laboring woman has shown no abnormalities during prenatal care, and when her delivery is attended by trained individuals."[20]

The acceptance of the obstetric specialist and the near elimination of the midwife have not solved the problem of the high infant mortality rate in the United States. While it is true that this rate declined from 124 deaths per 1,000 live births in 1910 to 18.5 in 1972, this country still lags behind many European countries which use midwives and nurse-midwives as integral parts of their health teams. In 1972, for example, Sweden (10.8), the Netherlands (11.7), Norway (11.8), Denmark (12.2), and England and Wales (17.2) all reported infant mortality rates below that of the United States. In fact, fifteen modern industrial nations reported infant mortality rates lower than that of the United States in 1972.[21]

Efforts to reduce the maternal mortality rate of the United States have proved more successful. During the mid-1930s, the maternal death rate began a precipitous decline. By the early 1960s, the United States was listed as one of the low maternal mortality countries, along with Denmark, England, Norway, and Sweden. The 1964 maternal death rate for the United States was 3.3 per 10,000 live births. By 1973, this figure had been reduced to 1.5. Nevertheless, there are certain European countries, including Denmark, Norway, and Sweden, whose rates are close to 0 per 10,000 live births.[22]

It is interesting to note how the health care programs of those European countries with maternal and infant mortality rates below that of the United States differ from the American way of health care. Three major distinctions are readily apparent. First, each of these countries has extensive government-sponsored insurance programs. In contrast, medical care in the United States is, for the

most part, privately financed. Second, European physicians employ more conservative obstetric practices than their American
counterparts. The frequency of forceps deliveries, cesarean sections, and the use of anesthesia during childbirth is much greater in
the United States than in Europe. Third, midwives and nurse-
midwives play important roles in European health care programs.
In 1963, for instance, midwives and student midwives attended
81 percent of all births in England and Wales. Most normal deliveries
in Sweden are assisted by midwives. In the Netherlands, where the
majority of births occur at home, the midwife also plays a major
role in the birth process.[23]

It is unfortunate that Americans have been so reluctant to endorse the concept of the midwife. It is quite likely that the present
infant and maternal mortality rates of the United States would
compare more favorably with other modern industrial nations if
properly educated midwives and nurse-midwives were utilized to
their fullest extent. The educating and training of midwives is certainly not the only way to bring about a reduction in the maternal
and infant mortality rates in the United States. It is, however, a
major step in the right direction.[24]

NOTES

1. Grace L. Meigs, *Maternal Mortality From All Conditions Connected
With Childbirth in the United States and Certain Other Countries*, United
States Department of Labor, Children's Bureau Publication, No. 19 (Wash-
ington, D.C., 1917), p. 7.

2. Rosemary Stevens, *American Medicine and the Public Interest* (New
Haven, Conn., 1971), p. 145.

3. Wilson H. Grabill, Clyde V. Kiser, and Pascal K. Whelpton, *The
Fertility of American Women* (New York, 1958), p. 27.

4. Research Committee of the American College of Nurse-Midwives,
Descriptive Data: Nurse-Midwives—U.S.A. (New York, [1972]), p. 6.

5. Suzanne Arms, *Immaculate Deception: A New Look at Women
and Childbirth in America* (Boston, 1975), pp. 51-86; Marion Sousa, *Childbirth at Home* (New York, 1977), pp. 21-51; Boston Women's Health
Collective, *Our Bodies, Ourselves: A Book By and For Women* (New York,
1976), pp. 267-270, 278-289. See also Program Notes, Rhode Island Women's Health Conference, Providence, R.I., March 27, 1976.

6. *Association for Childbirth at Home: Goals and Purposes* (Cerritos, Calif., 1976); *Home Oriented Maternity Experience: A Comprehensive Guide to Home Birth* (Washington, D.C., 1976), pp. 20-21; "Our Home-birth History," *Mothering*, 2 ([1976]), 78; *NAPSAC Statement of Purpose* (Chapel Hill, N.C., [1976]).

Of course, critics of hospital birth practices do not necessarily support the home childbirth movement. For example, the International Childbirth Education Association (ICEA), which has worked for several decades for the establishment of family-centered maternity and infant care, has declined to take an official position regarding the home childbirth issue. In 1976, after an emotionally charged two-hour discussion, the ICEA Board of Directors passed a resolution supporting the position "that childbirth education be available to all persons who desire or require it, irrespective of their plans for method or location of birth." Jamie Bolane, "ICEA Today," *ICEA News*, 15 (Fall 1976), 1. One of the most well-known critics of American hospital birth procedures is Doris B. Haire, former president of ICEA. See, for example, Doris B. Haire, *The Cultural Warping of Childbirth* (Seattle, Wash., 1972).

7. Information about physicians who support home childbirth can be found in the following: James D. Brew, "An Obstetrician's Point of View," in Charlotte and Fred Ward, *The Home Birth Book* (Washington, D.C., 1976), pp. 35-42; Mayer Eisenstein, "Homebirths and the Physician," in David Stewart and Lee Stewart, eds., *Safe Alternatives in Childbirth* (Chapel Hill, N.C., 1976), pp. 67-72; "The American College of Home Obstetrics," in Stewart and Stewart, *Safe Alternatives*, p. 183.

8. Lester Dessez Hazell, *Commonsense Childbirth* (New York, 1976), p. 145.

9. Arms, *Immaculate*, p. 156; Hazell, *Commonsense*, p. 144; *Home Oriented Maternity Experience*, p. 20; Shirley Streshinsky, "Are You Safer with a Midwife?" *Ms.* 2 (October 1973), 24-27; Sousa, *Childbirth*, p. 96.

10. "American College of Nurse-Midwives: Position on Home Births," *Journal of Nurse-Midwifery*, 19 (Spring 1974), 36. See also Irene Matousek, "Home Births—Myths and Message," *Journal of Nurse-Midwifery*, 19 (Spring 1974), 23-29.

11. "Letters to the Editor," *Journal of Nurse-Midwifery*, 20 (Spring 1975), 6; Charlotte Theriault Houde, "Issues in Nurse-Midwifery Education," *Journal of Nurse-Midwifery*, 20 (Fall 1975), 14. See also Ruth M. White, "A Nurse-Midwife Looks Ahead," *Journal of Nurse-Midwifery*, 19 (Fall 1974), 5.

12. "A State by State Rundown on Midwife Licensing Requirements," *Mothering*, 2 ([1976]), 62-63.

13. Streshinsky, "Are You Safer," 25. An interview with a Georgia

"granny" who has been attending births since 1918 was published in the *Atlanta Constitution*, October 31, 1975, 12D.

14. Arms, *Immaculate*, pp. 165-181; Hazell, *Commonsense*, pp. 29-40, 144-145; Sousa, *Childbirth*, pp. 118-120; Ward, *Home Birth Book*, pp. 47-52. Raven Lang, *Birth Book* (Palo Alto, Calif., 1972) and Ina May, *Spiritual Midwifery* (Summertown, Tenn., 1975) contain detailed descriptions of the experiences of contemporary lay midwives.

15. Florence Ellen Lee and Jay H. Glasser, "Role of Lay Midwifery in Maternity Care in a Large Metropolitan Area," *Public Health Reports*, 89 (November-December 1974), 538; Katherine Stanwick, "Welcome to Our Home . . . Helping Parents Learn About Birth," *Mothering*, 2 ([1976]), 82-85.

16. "A State by State Rundown on Midwife Licensing Requirements," 62; Fran Ventre, "The Making of a Legalized Lay Midwife," *Birth and the Family Journal*, 3 (Fall 1976), 109-115.

17. Sousa, *Childbirth*, pp. 96-97; Arms, *Immaculate*, pp. 179, 217-219. The arrests of the Santa Cruz midwives forced the California courts to consider whether attending births constituted the same thing as practicing medicine. The question of the legality of lay midwifery in California had not been clarified as of July 1976. "A State by State Rundown on Midwife Licensing Requirements," 63; George J. Annas, "Legal Aspects of Homebirth and Other Childbirth Alternatives," in Stewart and Stewart, *Safe Alternatives*, pp. 167-168; Jackie Christeve, "Midwives Busted in Santa Cruz," *Second Wave*, 3 (Summer 1974), 5-10; Karen Hope Ehrlich, "The Santa Cruz Birth Center Today," *Birth and the Family Journal*, 3 (Fall 1976), 119-126; Michael Goldberg, "California Birth Center Busted," *Rough Times*, 4 (March-May 1974), 4; "Midwives Busted," *Off Our Backs*, 4 (June 1974), 8.

18. *First International Conference of Practicing Midwives* (El Paso, Tex. [1976]), 15; "You Mean We Still Have Midwives?" *Mothering*, 2 ([1976]), 61-62; Arlyn Macdonald, "Impressions—First International Conference of Practicing Midwives," *Mothering*, 3 ([1977]), 52-59. Interview with conference participant, Adele Alexandre, Providence, R. I., January 20, 1977. See also Fran Ventre, "Proposal for Education of Certified Midwives" (mimeographed, Washington, D.C., 1976).

19. Midwives from the The Farm in Summertown, Tenn., began publishing a newsletter, *The Practicing Midwife*, early in 1977. Similarly, midwife proponents from Vermont and New Hampshire began publishing a newsletter, *Midwife to Midwife*, early in 1977.

20. Lewis E. Mehl and Gail H. Peterson, "Management of the Complications of Home Delivery: An Analysis of Results from the Santa Cruz Birth Center, California," in Sousa, *Childbirth*, pp. 180, 194-196, passim. See

also Lewis E. Mehl, "Statistical Outcomes of Homebirths in the United States," in Stewart and Stewart, *Safe Alternatives*, pp. 73-100; Lewis E. Mehl, Gail H. Peterson, Nancy S. Shaw, and Don C. Creevy, "Complications of Home Birth," *Birth and the Family Journal*, 2 (Fall-Winter 1975), 123-131; Lewis E. Mehl, "Home Delivery Research Today—A Review," *Women and Health*, 1 (September-October 1976), 3-11; Lester Dessez Hazell, *Birth Goes Home* (Seattle, Wash., 1974); Arms, *Immaculate*, pp. 182-192.

21. United States Bureau of the Census, *Statistical Abstract of the United States: 1975* (Washington, D.C., 1975), p. 63; *United Nations Demographic Yearbook, 1974* (New York, 1975); Helen M. Wallace and Hyman Goldstein, "The Status of Infant Mortality in Sweden and the United States," *Journal of Pediatrics*, 87 (December 1975), 995.

22. Sam Shapiro, Edward R. Schlesinger, and Robert E. L. Nesbitt, Jr., *Infant, Perinatal, Maternal and Childhood Mortality in the United States* (Cambridge, Mass., 1968), pp. 145, 158; *Statistical Abstract of the United States: 1975*, p. 63.

In recent years, much discussion has ensued concerning the high mortality rate among nonwhite infants and mothers. See, for example, Eleanor P. Hunt, *Recent Demographic Trends and Their Effects on Maternal and Child Health Needs and Services*, United States Department of Health, Education and Welfare, Children's Bureau Publication (Washington, D.C., 1966), p. 9; Eleanor P. Hunt and Alice D. Chenoweth, "Recent Trends in Infant Mortality in the United States," *American Journal of Public Health*, 51 (February 1961), 190; Shapiro, Schlesinger, and Nesbitt, *Infant*, pp. 23, 162. During the 1915-1919 period, nonwhite maternal deaths occurred 1.79 times more often than white maternal deaths. By the early 1960s, nonwhite women had four times the maternal mortality rate found among white women. In 1970, this figure had been slightly reduced to 3.9. Nevertheless, the overall rate of decline for whites and nonwhites has been much more even. From 1915 to 1970, the white maternal mortality rate declined by 98 percent and the nonwhite rate declined by 96 percent. The excess of nonwhite infant deaths to white deaths is not so great. During the 1915-1919 period, nonwhite infant deaths occurred 1.5 times more often than white deaths. By the early 1960s nonwhite infants had 1.8 times the infant mortality found among white infants. In 1970, this figure had been slightly reduced to 1.7. Moreover, from 1915 to 1970, the white infant mortality rate declined by 81 percent, and the nonwhite rate declined by 79 percent. United States Bureau of the Census, *Vital Statistics of the United States, 1970* (Washington, D.C., 1974).

23. Helen C. Chase, "Perinatal and Infant Mortality in the United States and Six West European Countries," *American Journal of Public Health*,

57 (October 1967), 1744-1746; Macy Foundation, *The Training and Responsibilities of the Midwife* (New York, 1967), pp. 70, 88; Wallace and Goldstein, "Status," 997; Arms, *Immaculate*, pp. 270-291.

24. See, for example, Barry S. Levy, Frederick S. Wilkinson, and William M. Marine, "Reducing Neonatal Mortality Rate with Nurse-Midwives," *American Journal of Obstetrics and Gynecology*, 109 (January 1971), 50-58; Lillian Runnerstrom, "The Effectiveness of Nurse-Midwifery in a Supervised Hospital Environment," *Bulletin of the American College of Nurse-Midwives*, 14 (May 1969), 40-52; Marie C. Meglen and Helen V. Burst, "Nurse-Midwives Make a Difference," *Nursing Outlook*, 22 (June 1974), 386-389; Lee and Glasser, "Role of Lay Midwifery," 537-544.

Bibliography

PRIMARY SOURCES

Books and Pamphlets

An Appeal to the Medical Society of Rhode-Island, in Behalf of Woman to be Restored to her Natural Rights as "Midwife" and Elevated by Education to be the Physician of her Own Sex. Printed for the Author. 1851.

Arms, Suzanne. *Immaculate Deception: A New Look at Women and Childbirth in America.* Boston: Houghton Mifflin, 1975.

Association for Childbirth at Home: Goals and Purposes. Cerritos, Calif., 1976.

Austin, George Lowell. *Perils of American Women, or a Doctor's Talk with Maiden, Wife and Mother.* Boston: Lee & Shepard, 1883.

Baker, S. Josephine. *Child Hygiene.* New York: Harper & Brothers, Publishers, 1925.

Baker, S. Josephine. *Fighting for Life.* New York: Macmillan Company, 1939.

Bard, Samuel. *Compendium of the Theory and Practice of Midwifery.* New York: Collins, 1807.

Bean, Constance A. *Labor & Delivery: An Observer's Diary.* Garden City, N.Y.: Doubleday & Company, Inc., 1977.

Berkeley, Comyns. *A Handbook for Midwives and Maternity Nurses.* London: Cassell & Company, 1909.

Billings, John S., and Henry M. Hurd. *Hospitals, Dispensaries and Nursing.* Baltimore: The Johns Hopkins University Press, 1894.

Blackwell, Elizabeth. *Essays in Medical Sociology.* London: Ernest Bell, 1902.

Blackwell, Elizabeth. *Pioneer Work in Opening the Medical Profession to Women.* London: Longman's Green & Company, 1895.

Breckinridge, Mary. *Wide Neighborhoods: A Story of the Frontier Nursing Service.* New York: Harper & Brothers, Publishers, 1952.

Brown, Dorothy Kirchwey. *The Case for Acceptance of the Sheppard-Towner Act.* Washington, D.C.: National League of Women Voters, 1923.

Calder, A. B. *Lectures on Midwifery for Midwives.* New York: William Wood & Company, 1905.

Channing, Walter. *Remarks on the Employment of Females as Practitioners in Midwifery.* Boston: Cummings & Hilliard, 1820.

Chavasse, Pye Henry. *Woman as a Wife and Mother.* Philadelphia: W. B. Evans, 1870.

Commander, Lydia. *The American Idea.* New York: A. S. Barnes & Company, 1907.

Conant, Clarence M. *An Obstetric Mentor. A Handbook of Homeopathic Treatment Required during Pregnancy, Parturition and the Puerperal Season.* New York: A. L. Chatterton, 1884.

De Lee, Joseph B. *The Principles and Practice of Obstetrics.* Philadelphia: W. B. Saunders, 1934.

Drake, Emma F. Anzell. *Maternity Without Suffering.* Philadelphia: The Vir Publishing Company, 1902.

Drake, Emma F. Anzell. *What a Young Wife Ought to Know.* Philadelphia: The Vir Publishing Company, 1901.

Dye, John H. *Painless Childbirth; or Healthy Mothers and Healthy Children.* Silver Creek, N.Y.: Brown, Elliott & Spears, 1884.

Education for Nurse-Midwifery: The Report of the Second Work Conference on Nurse-Midwifery Education. New York: Maternity Center Association, 1967.

Education for Nurse-Midwifery: The Report of the Work Conference on Nurse-Midwifery. New York: American College of Nurse-Midwifery, 1958.

Fiftieth Annual Report of the Maternity Center Association, 1918-1968. New York: Maternity Center Association, [1969].

First International Conference of Practicing Midwives. El Paso, Tex., [1976].

Flexner, Abraham. *Medical Education in the United States and Canada: A Report to the Carnegie Foundation for the Advancement of Teaching.* Bulletin No. 4. Boston: P. B. Updike, 1910.

Forman, Alice M. *Patterns of Legislation and the Practice of Nurse-Midwifery in the U.S.A.* New York: American College of Nurse-Midwives, 1974.

Forman, Alice M., Susan H. Fischman, and Lucille Woodville, eds. *New Horizons in Midwifery.* Proceedings of the 16th Triennial Congress of the International Confederation of Midwives, October 28-November 3, 1972. Baltimore: Waverly Press, 1973.

Forty-Fifth Annual Report and Log, 1915-1963, of the Maternity Center Association. New York: Maternity Center Association, [1964].

Fothergill, W. E. *Manual of Midwifery for the Use of Students and Practitioners.* New York: MacMillan & Company, 1896.

Frankel, Lee K. *The Present Status of Maternal and Infant Hygiene in the United States.* New York: Metropolitan Life Insurance Company, 1927.

Fullerton, Anna M. *A Handbook of Obstetrical Nursing for Nurses, Students and Mothers.* Philadelphia: P. Blakiston, Son & Company, 1890.

Galabin, Alfred L. *A Manual of Midwifery.* Philadelphia: P. Blakiston, Son & Company, 1886.

Galdston, Iago. *Maternal Deaths—The Ways to Prevention.* New York: The Commonwealth Fund, 1937.

Garrigues, Henry J. *Practical Guide in Antiseptic Midwifery in Hospitals and Private Practice.* Detroit: G. S. Davis, 1886.

Geffen, Dennis. *Public Health and Social Services: Elementary Text for Midwives.* London: Edward Arnold & Company, 1940.

Glisan, Rodney. *Textbook of Modern Midwifery.* Philadelphia: Presley Blakiston, 1881.

Goldman, Emma. *Living My Life,* 2 vols. Reprint of 1931 edition. New York: Dover Publications, Inc., 1970.

Harland, Marion. *Eve's Daughters: or Common Sense for Maid, Wife and Mother.* New York: John R. Anderson & Henry S. Allen, 1882.

Hazell, Lester Dessez. *Birth Goes Home.* Seattle, Wash.: Catalyst Publishing Company, 1974.

Hazell, Lester Dessez. *Commonsense Childbirth.* New York: Berkley Publishing Corporation, 1976.

Herb, Ferdinand. *Beauty and Motherhood.* Chicago: Medico Press, 1915.

Holbrook, M. L. *Parturition Without Pain: A Code of Directions for Escaping the Primal Curse.* 15th edition. New York: M. L. Holbrook, 1891.

Hollick, Frederick. *The Matron's Manual of Midwifery and the Diseases of Women during Pregnancy and in Child Bed.* 47th edition. New York: T. W. Strong, 1848.

Hollick, Frederick. *The Origin of Life and Process of Reproduction in Plants and Animals, with the Anatomy and Physiology of the Human Generative System, Male and Female, and the Causes, Prevention and Cure of the Special Diseases to Which It is Liable.* Philadelphia: David McKay, 1878.

Home Oriented Maternity Experience: A Comprehensive Guide to Home Birth. Washington, D.C.: HOME, Inc., 1976.

Hooker, Ransom S. *Maternal Mortality in New York City: A Study of*

All Puerperal Deaths, 1930-1932. New York: The Commonwealth Fund, 1933.

Hoover, Herbert. *The Memoirs of Herbert Hoover, the Cabinet and the Presidency, 1920-1933.* New York: Macmillan Company, 1952.

Hunt, Harriot K. *Glances and Glimpses.* Reprint of 1856 edition. New York: Source Book Press, 1970.

Jewett, Charles. *Outlines of Obstetrics: A Syllabus of Lectures Delivered at the Long Island College Hospital.* Philadelphia: W. B. Saunders, 1894.

Joint Study Group of the International Federation of Gynecology and Obstetrics and the International Confederation of Midwives. *Maternity Care in the World: International Survey of Midwifery Practice and Training.* Oxford, England: Pergamon Press Ltd., 1966.

Kitzinger, Sheila. *The Experience of Childbirth.* Middlesex, England: Penguin Books, Ltd., 1974.

Knopf, Sigard Adolphus. *An Open Letter on Maternal Mortality to Dr. George W. Kosmak.* New York, 1932.

Kucher, Joseph. *Puerperal Convalescence and the Diseases of the Puerperal Period.* New York: J. H. Vail & Company, 1886.

Lang, Raven. *Birth Book.* Palo Alto, Calif.: Genesis Press, 1972.

Leishman, William. *A System of Midwifery, Including the Diseases of Pregnancy and the Puerperal State.* 3rd American edition. Philadelphia: H. C. Lea, 1879.

Lusk, W. T. *The Science and Art of Midwifery.* New York: D. Appleton & Company, 1882.

Lyman, Eliza Barton. *The Coming Woman: or the Royal Road to Perfection.* Lansing, Mich.: W. S. George, 1880.

Macy Foundation. *The Midwife in the United States.* New York: Josiah Macy, Jr., Foundation, 1968.

Macy Foundation. *The Training and Responsibilities of the Midwife.* New York: Josiah Macy, Jr., Foundation, 1967.

Marsden, J. H. *Hand-book of Practical Midwifery, Including Full Instructions for the Homeopathic Treatment of the Disorders of Pregnancy and the Accidents and Diseases Incident to Labor and the Puerperal State.* New York: Boericke & Tafel, 1879.

Maternity Center Association. *Public Health Nursing in Obstetrics.* New York: Maternity Center Association, 1943.

Maternity Center Association. *Twenty Years of Nurse-Midwifery, 1933-1953.* New York: Maternity Center Association, [1955].

May, Ina. *Spiritual Midwifery.* Summertown, Tenn.: The Book Publishing Company, 1975.

Meadows, Alfred. *A Manual of Midwifery*. Philadelphia: Lindsay & Blakiston, 1871.

Medical Care for the American People: The Final Report of the Committee on the Costs of Medical Care. Chicago: University of Chicago Press, 1932.

Mitchell, S. Weir. *Doctor and Patient*. Philadelphia: J. B. Lippincott Company, 1904.

Mosher, Clelia Duel. *Health and the Woman Movement*. 2nd revised edition. New York: Woman Press, 1918.

Mosher, Clelia Duel. *Woman's Physical Freedom*. 3rd revised edition. New York: Woman Press, 1923.

Napheys, George H. *The Physical Life of Woman: Advice to the Maiden, Wife, and Mother*. Philadelphia: David McKay, 1890.

NAPSAC Statement of Purpose. Chapel Hill, N.C., [1976].

Nicholson, William R. *An Anachronism of the Twentieth Century: The Midwife*. Nathan Lewis Hatfield Lectures. [Philadelphia, 1921].

Nihell, Elizabeth. *A Treatise on the Art of Midwifery. Setting Forth Various Abuses therein, especially as to the practice with Instruments: the Whole serving to put all Rational Inquirers in a fair way of very safely forming their own Judgment upon the Question: which it is best to employ, In Cases of Pregnancy and Lying-In, a Man-Midwife or, a Midwife*. London: Morley, 1760.

Partridge, Edward L. *A Manual of Obstetrics*. New York: William Wood & Company, 1884.

Patterns of Legislation and the Practice of Nurse-Midwifery in the United States. New York: American College of Nurse-Midwives, 1974.

Peacock, Gladys Marcia. *I Wanted to Live in America*. Lexington, Ky.: Frontier Nursing Service, 1942.

Philadelphia County Medical Society Committee on Maternal Welfare. *Maternal Mortality in Philadelphia, 1931-1933*. Philadelphia: Philadelphia County Medical Society, 1934.

Playfair School of Midwifery: Annual Announcement, 1899. Chicago, 1899.

Playfair, W. S. *A Treatise on the Science and Practice of Midwifery*. 3rd American edition. Philadelphia: H. C. Lea, 1880.

Reed, Louis S. *Midwives, Chiropodists and Optometrists: Their Place in Medical Care*. No. 15, Publications of the Committee on the Costs of Medical Care. Chicago: University of Chicago Press, 1932.

Reed, Mary L. *The Mothercraft Manual*. Boston: Little, Brown & Company, 1917.

Report of the Committee of the New York Obstetrical Society to Review the Maternal Mortality Report of the Public Health Relations Committee of the New York Academy of Medicine. New York: Paul B. Hoeber, 1934.

Research Committee of the American College of Nurse-Midwives. *Descriptive Data: Nurse-Midwives—U.S.A.* New York: American College of Nurse-Midwives, [1972].

Research Division of the American Child Health Association. *A Health Survey of 86 Cities.* New York: American Child Health Association, 1925.

Reynolds, Edward, and Franklin S. Newell. *Practical Obstetrics: A Text-Book for Practitioners and Students.* Philadelphia: Lea Brothers & Company, 1902.

Rosenberg, Charles, and Carroll Smith-Rosenberg, eds. *The Male Midwife and the Female Doctor: The Gynecology Controversy in Nineteenth-Century America.* New York: Arno Press, 1974.

Sanger, Margaret. *An Autobiography.* Reprint of 1938 edition. New York: Dover Publications, Inc., 1971.

Saur, Prudence B. *Maternity: A Book for Every Wife and Mother.* Chicago: L. P. Miller, 1891.

Schmalhausen, S. D., and V. F. Calverton, eds. *Woman's Coming of Age.* New York: Horace Liveright, Inc., 1931.

Scovil, Elizabeth R. *Preparation for Motherhood.* Philadelphia: Henry Altimus, 1896.

Seaman, Valentine. *The Midwives' Monitor, and Mother's Mirror.* New York: Collins, 1800.

Slemons, Josiah Morris. *The Prospective Mother: A Handbook for Women During Pregnancy.* New York: D. Appleton & Company, 1912.

Sousa, Marion. *Childbirth at Home.* New York: Bantam Books, 1977.

Standards for Maternity Care. Prepared by the Committee on Maternity Care of the Children's Welfare Federation and a Committee Appointed by the New York Obstetrical Society. New York: The Children's Welfare Federation, 1930.

Stevens, Margaret. *Woman and Marriage.* New York: Frederick A. Stokes Company, 1910.

Stewart, David, and Lee Stewart, eds. *Safe Alternatives in Childbirth.* Chapel Hill, N.C.: NAPSAC, 1976.

Stockham, Alice B. *Tokology: A Book for Every Woman.* Chicago: Sanitary Publishing Company, 1885.

Thomas, T. Gaillard. *A Practical Treatise on the Diseases of Women.* Philadelphia: Henry C. Lea's Sons & Company, 1880.

United Nations Demographic Yearbook, 1974. New York: United Nations, 1975.

Van Blarcom, Carolyn Conant. *The Midwife in England: Being a Study in England of the Working of the English Midwives Act of 1902.* Philadelphia: William F. Fell Company, 1913.

Verdi, Tullio Suzzara. *Maternity: A Popular Treatise for Young Wives and Mothers.* Philadelphia: F. E. Boeriche, 1885.

Vietor, Agnes C., ed. *A Woman's Quest: The Life of Marie E. Zakrzewska.* New York: D. Appleton & Company, 1924.

Ward, Charlotte and Fred. *The Home Birth Book.* Washington, D.C.: INSCAPE Publishers, 1976.

Ways of Woman in Their Physical, Moral, and Intellectual Relations. By a medical man. New York: J. P. Jewett, 1873.

What Is a Nurse-Midwife? New York: American College of Nurse-Midwives, 1973.

White House Conference on Child Health and Protection. *Fetal, Newborn, and Maternal Mortality and Morbidity.* New York: The Century Company, 1933.

White House Conference on Child Health and Protection, 1930: Addresses and Abstracts of Committee Reports. New York: The Century Company, 1931.

White House Conference on Child Health and Protection. *Obstetric Education.* New York: The Century Company, 1932.

White House Conference on Child Health and Protection. *Public Health Organization.* New York: The Century Company, 1932.

Willeford, Mary Bristow. *Income and Health in Remote Rural Areas: A Study of 400 Families in Leslie County, Kentucky.* New York: [n.p.], 1932.

Williams, J. Whitridge. *Obstetrics: A Textbook for the Use of Students and Practitioners.* New York: D. Appleton & Company, 1903.

Wollstonecraft, Mary. *A Vindication of the Rights of Woman.* Reprint of 1792 edition. New York: W. W. Norton, 1967.

Woman's Work in the Field of Medicine. New York: The College of Midwifery, 1883.

Periodicals

American Journal of Nursing. 12 (1912)-46 (1946).
American Journal of Public Health. 1 (1911)-20 (1930).
American Midwife. 1 (November 1895)-2 (October 1896).
Birth and the Family Journal. 1 (1973-1974)-3 (1976).

Journal of the American Medical Association. 38 (1897)-105 (1935).

Journal of the Maine Medical Association. 3 (1912)-20 (1930).

Journal of Nurse-Midwifery. 1 (1956)-21 (1976).

Medical Woman's Journal. 1 (1893)-37 (1930).

Mothering. 1-2 ([1976])-3 ([1977]).

Nurse-Midwife Bulletin. 1 (May 1954)-2 October 1955).

Public Health Nursing. 3 (1911)-35 (1943).

Topics of Interest to Midwives. 2 (January 1918)-3 (February 1918).

Transactions of the American Association for the Study and Prevention of Infant Mortality. 1 (1910)-8 (1917).

Transactions of the American Child Health Association. 1 (1923)-6 (1929).

Transactions of the American Child Hygiene Association. 9 (1918)-13 (1922).

Women and Health. 1 (1976).

Articles

Abbott, Grace. "The Midwife in Chicago." *American Journal of Sociology,* 20 (March 1915), 684-699.

Adair, Fred L. "Mortality Associated with Maternity." *American Journal of Obstetrics and Gynecology,* 68 (July 1954), 20-28.

Allport, Walter H. "Relation of the Community to the Midwife." *Chicago Medical Recorder,* 34 (1912), 123-131.

Alsop, Gulielma. "The Right to Be Well Born." *Woman Citizen,* 8 (February 1924), 30.

"Aunt Sarah: Tennessee's Champion Midwife." *Newsweek,* 48 (August 1956), 54.

Bailey, Harold. "Control of Midwives." *American Journal of Obstetrics and Gynecology,* 6 (September 1923), 293-298.

Baker, S. Josephine. "Getting the Right Start." *Ladies' Home Journal,* 47 (August 1930), 80.

Baker, S. Josephine. "High Cost of Babies." *Ladies' Home Journal,* 40 (October 1923), 13, 212-213.

Baker, S. Josephine. "Reduction of Infant Mortality in New York City." *American Journal of the Diseases of Children,* 5 (February 1913), 151-161.

Baker, S. Josephine. "Schools for Midwives." *American Journal of Obstetrics and the Diseases of Women and Children,* 65 (1912), 256-270.

Baker, S. Josephine. "Why Do Our Mothers and Babies Die?" *Ladies' Home Journal,* 39 (April 1922), 39, 174.

Baldy, J. M. "Is the Midwife a Necessity?" *American Journal of Obstetrics and the Diseases of Women and Children*, 73 (March 1916), 399-407.

Baughman, Greer. "A Preliminary Report Upon the Midwife Situation in Virginia." *Virginia Medical Monthly*, 54 (March 1928), 749-750.

Bayley, Mary E. "The Prospective Mother." *Delineator*, 99 (September 1921), 30.

Beitler, F. V. "Reduction of Infant Mortality Due to Prenatal and Obstetrical Conditions." *American Journal of Obstetrics and the Diseases of Women and Children*, 77 (1918), 481-484.

Bergland, J. McF. "Changes in Obstetrical Procedure During the Last Thirty-Five Years." *Southern Medical Journal*, 32 (1939), 187-191.

Bigelow, H. A. "Maternity Care in Rural Areas by Public Health Nurses." *American Journal of Public Health*, 27 (October 1937), 975-980.

Bird, Aldine R. "Progress of Obstetric Knowledge in America." *Hygenia*, 11 (May 1933), 437-439.

Blankenship, M. Beatrice. "Enduring Miracle." *Atlantic*, 152 (October 1933), 409-415.

Bolane, Jamie. "ICEA Today." *ICEA News*, 15 (Fall 1976), 1.

Bowdoin, Joe P. "The Midwife Problem." *Transactions of the Section on Preventive Medicine and Public Health of the American Medical Association* (1928), 90-95.

Bradley, Frances Sage. "Save the Country Baby." *Survey*, 51 (December 1923), 321-323.

Bradley, Frances Sage. "Which—A Well Baby or a Boyish Form?" *Hygenia*, 5 (June 1927), 298-299.

Breckinridge, Mary. "An Adventure in Midwifery." *Survey*, 57 (October 1926), 25-27, 47.

Breckinridge, Mary. "Hard-Riding Nurses of Kentucky." *Literary Digest*, 96 (March 1928), 29-30.

Breckinridge, Mary. "Maternity in the Mountains." *North American Review*, 226 (December 1928), 765-768.

Breckinridge, Mary. "Midwifery in the Kentucky Mountains, An Investigation in 1923." *Quarterly Bulletin of the Frontier Nursing Service*, 17 (Spring 1942), 29-53.

Breckinridge, Mary. "Where the Frontier Lingers." *Rotarian*, 47 (September 1935), 9-12, 50.

Brickner, Ruth. "Making the Most of Maternity." *Parents' Magazine*, 12 (March 1937), 27, 67-71.

Brocon, Charlotte B. "Obstetric Practice Among the Chinese in San Francisco." *Pacific Medical and Surgical Journal*, 26 (July 1883), 15-21.

Browne, Helen E., and Gertrude Isaacs. "The Frontier Nursing Service:

The Primary Care Nurse in the Community Hospital." *American Journal of Obstetrics and Gynecology*, 124 (January 1976), 14-17.

Buchman, A. P. "Faulty Midwifery and Its Relations to Gynecology." *Obstetric Gazette*, 3 (1880), 62-66.

Buckle, L. "Acted as Her Own Midwife." *West Virginia Medical Journal*, 6 (April 1912), 343.

Burnett, John E. "A Physician-Sponsored Community Nurse-Midwife Program." *Obstetrics and Gynecology*, 40 (November 1972), 719-723.

Butler, Mary L. "Early History of Maternal Associations." *Chautauguan*, 31 (May 1900), 38-42.

Chapin, Charles V. "The Control of Midwifery." *Medical Progress*, 39 (April 1923), 76-79.

Chesterton, G. K. "Maternity and Child Welfare." *New Statesman*, 13 (May 1919), 116.

"Childbirth Aids." *Time*, 32 (October 1938), 37.

"Childbirth: Nature vs. Drugs." *Time*, 2 (May 1936), 32, 34, 38.

Clark, Taliaferro. "Training of Midwives." *Chicago Medical Recorder*, 46 (1924), 297-304.

Cody, Edmund F. "The Registered Midwife: A Necessity." *Boston Medical and Surgical Journal*, 168 (March 1913), 416-418.

Collins, Frederick L. "Expectant Mothers and Fathers." *Ladies' Home Journal*, 48 (January 1931), 23, 101-103.

Comstock, Sarah. "Mothercraft: A New Profession for Women." *Good Housekeeping*, 59 (December 1914), 672-678.

Corbin, Hazel. "An Adequate Local Maternity Program." *Proceedings of the National Conference of Social Work*, (1924), 248-252.

Corson, Hiram. "Thoughts on Midwifery." *Medical and Surgical Reporter*, 40 (January 1879), 3-5.

Costill, Henry B. "Midwifery Supervision Succeeds in New Jersey." *Nation's Health*, 8 (April 1926), 255-257.

"Country Doctor Writes a Letter: Needless Maternal Mortality." *Ladies' Home Journal*, 54 (May 1937), 4.

Crowell, F. Elisabeth. "The Midwives of New York." *Charities and the Commons*, 17 (January 1907), 667-677.

Crumpler, Paul. "The Midwife." *Charlotte (North Carolina) Medical Journal*, 73 (1916), 159-160.

Darlington, Thomas. "The Present Status of the Midwife." *American Journal of Obstetrics and the Diseases of Women and Children*, 63 (1911), 870-884.

Davis, Clara M. "Obstetrical Service for the Laboring Classes and the Relation of the Midwife to It in Michigan." *Journal of the Michigan State Medical Society*, 7 (May 1908), 213-218.

Davis, Marine. "Childbirth." *Pictorial Review*, 40 (October 1938), 18-19, 66-67.

"Death Rate Among Mothers." *Commonweal*, 19 (December 1933), 143-144.

De Kruif, Paul. "Forgotten Mothers." *Ladies' Home Journal*, 53 (December 1936), 12-13, 64, 66, 68.

De Kruif, Paul. "Saver of Mothers." *Ladies' Home Journal*, 49 (March 1932), 6-7, 124-125.

De Kruif, Paul. "Why Should Mothers Die?" *Ladies' Home Journal*, 53 (March 1936), 8-9, 103-108.

De Lee, Joseph B. "Before the Baby Comes." *Delineator*, 109 (October 1926), 35, 84.

De Lee, Joseph B. "The Prophylactic Forceps Operation." *American Journal of Obstetrics and Gynecology*, 1 (1920), 34-44.

"Discussion on Proposed Legislation Against Midwives." *Medical Record*, 53 (February 1898), 210-211.

"Doctor Studies Effects of Pain-Killing Drugs." *News-Week*, 9 (May 1937), 42.

Dunbar, Olivia. "To the Baby, Debtor." *Good Housekeeping*, 67 (November 1918), 35-36.

Earnshaw, G. F. "A Child Is to Be Born." *Hygenia*, 4 (August 1926), 445-447.

Eastman, Nicholsen J. "Whither American Obstetrics." *New England Journal of Medicine*, 224 (1941), 89-93.

Edgar, J. Clifton. "The Education, Licensing and Supervision of the Midwife." *American Journal of Obstetrics and the Diseases of Women and Children*, 73 (March 1916), 385-398.

Edgar, J. Clifton. "The Remedy for the Midwife Problem." *American Journal of Obstetrics and the Diseases of Women and Children*, 63 (1911), 881-884.

Edgar, J. Clifton. "Why the Midwife?" *American Journal of Obstetrics and the Diseases of Women and Children*, 77 (1918), 242-255.

Edgar, J. Clifton. "Why the Midwife?" *Transactions of the American Gynecological Society*, 43 (1918), 213-236.

"Editorial." *American Gynecological and Obstetrical Journal*, 7 (July 1895), 22-25.

Emmons, Arthur B., and James L. Huntington. "The Midwife: Her Future in the United States." *American Journal of Obstetrics and the Diseases of Women and Children*, 65 (March 1912), 393-404.

Emmons, Arthur B. and James L. Huntington. "A Review of the Midwife Situation." *Boston Medical and Surgical Journal*, 164 (1911), 251-262.

Eve, Robert C. "Licensing of Midwives." *Charlotte (North Carolina) Medical Journal*, 6 (1895), 990-995.

Fishbein, Morris. "The Costs of High Obstetrical Care." *American Mercury*, 30 (September 1933), 61-63.

Fletcher, Grace N. "Balancing the Baby Budget." *Century*, 89 (1925-1926), 419-425.

Folks, R. "Obstetrics in the Tenements." *Charities*, 9 (November 1902), 429-438.

Foote, J. A. "Legislative Measures Against Maternal and Infant Mortality." *American Journal of Obstetrics and the Diseases of Women and Children*, 80 (1919), 534-551.

"Frontier Nurse." *Literary Digest*, 124 (August 1937), 12.

Furnas, J. C. "That Mothers May Live." *Ladies' Home Journal*, 56 (November 1939), 21, 56-58.

Garrigues, H. J. "Midwives." *Medical News*, 72 (1898), 232-236.

Gewin, W. C. "Careless and Unscientific Midwifery with Special References to Some Features of the Work of Midwives." *Alabama Medical Journal*, 18 (1905-1906), 629-635.

Gold, Louis. "The Stork in New York." *American Mercury*, 32 (August 1934), 476-484.

Green, H. W. "Prenatal Instruction." *Proceedings of the National Conference of Social Work* (1927), 193-194.

Gwathmey, J. T. "Must Safe Childbirth Be Painful?" *Parents' Magazine*, 13 (February 1938), 22-23.

Halle, Rita S. "Make Motherhood Safe." *Good Housekeeping*, 98 (May 1934), 90, 233-238.

Hamilton, B. Wallace. "Before the Baby Arrives." *Delineator*, 93 (October 1918), 24.

"Handbook for Midwives." *American Journal of Obstetrics and the Diseases of Women and Children*, 6 (1873-1874), 700-701.

Hanson, Henry, and Lucile S. Blackly. "Present Status of Midwifery in Florida." *Southern Medical Journal*, 25 (December 1932), 1252-1258.

Hardin, E. R. "The Midwife Problem." *Southern Medical Journal*, 18 (1925), 347-350.

Hartley, E. C. and Ruth E. Boynton. "A Survey of the Midwife Situation in Minnesota." *Minnesota Medicine*, 7 (June 1924), 439-446.

Haynes, D. M. "The Vanishing Obstetrician." *Southern Medical Journal*, 61 (May 1968), 465-470.

"Hazards of Childbirth." *Nation*, 137 (November 1933), 612.

Hedger, Caroline. "Midwives and Blindness." *Illinois Medical Journal*, 21 (April 1912), 419-425.

Hellman, Louis, and Francis B. O'Brien, Jr. "Nurse-Midwifery—an Experiment in Maternity Care." *Obstetrics and Gynecology*, 24 (September 1964), 343-349.

Heusinkveld, Gerritt. "Training of Midwives." *Southwestern Medicine*, 18 (September 1934), 303-305.

Hill, T. J. "Some Remarks on the Midwifery Question: Must the Midwife Perish?" *Medical Record*, 4 (October 1898), 474-475.

Holmes, Rudolph W. "Midwife Practice: An Anachronism." *Illinois Medical Journal*, 37 (January 1920), 27-31.

Howard, William Travis, Jr. "The Real Risk Rate of Death to Mothers from Causes Connected with Childbirth." *American Journal of Hygiene*, (March 1921), 197-233.

Huntington, James L. "The Midwife in Massachusetts: Her Anomalous Position." *Boston Medical and Surgical Journal*, 168 (March 1913), 418-421.

Huntington, James L. "Midwives in Massachusetts." *Boston Medical and Surgical Journal*, 167 (October 1912), 542-548.

Huntington, James L. "The Pregnancy Clinic and the Midwife: A Comparison." *Boston Medical and Surgical Journal*, 173 (November 1915), 764-766.

Huntington, James L. "The Regulation of Midwifery." *Boston Medical and Surgical Journal*, 167 (1912), 84-87.

Husserl, S. "Necessity of the Scientific Training of Midwives." *Journal of the Medical Society of New Jersey*, 9 (December 1912), 349-351.

Hutchinson, Woods. "When the Stork Arrives." *Good Housekeeping*, 59 (July 1914), 100-103.

"Is the Twilight Sleep Safe—For Me?" *Woman's Home Companion*, 42 (January 1915), 10, 43.

Jarrett, Elizabeth. "The Midwife or the Woman Doctor." *Medical Record*, 54 (October 1898), 610-611.

Jeidell, Helmina, and Willa M. Fricke. "The Midwives of Anne Arundel County, Maryland." *Johns Hopkins Hospital Bulletin*, 23 (1912), 279-281.

Jones, I. W. "Childbirth With Less Pain and More Safety." *Parents' Magazine*, 8 (February 1933), 18-19.

Jordan, Philip. "Meeker Day on Midwifery." *Ohio Medical Journal*, 39 (1943), 1133-1134.

Kenyon, Josephine H. "Prenatal Care." *Good Housekeeping*, 103 (July 1936), 102.

Knox, J. H. Mason, Jr. "A Survey of Maternal Deaths in Maryland." *American Journal of Obstetrics and Gynecology*, 21 (1931), 143-147.

Kompert, G. "Midwives and their Disregard for Antiseptics." *Medical Record*, 53 (February 1898), 331.

Kortright, J. L. "Should Midwives be Registered?" *New York Journal of Gynecology and Obstetrics*, 3 (1893), 197-202.

Kortright, J. L. "Should Midwives be Registered?" *Transactions of the Medical Society of New York*, 18 (1893), 416-421.

Kosmak, George W. "Certain Aspects of the Midwife Problem in Relation to the Medical Profession and Community." *Medical Record,* 85 (June 1914), 1013-1017.

Kosmak George W. "The Midwife." *Briefs,* 8 (1944), 22-25.

Lapham, Anna Ross. "A Child Is to Be Born." *Hygenia,* 4 (September 1926), 514-517.

Lenroot, Katherine F. "Safety for Mothers." *Parents' Magazine,* 10 (May 1935), 15.

Leupp, Constance and Burton J. Hendrick. "Twilight Sleep in America." *McClure's,* 44 (April 1915), 25-37.

Levy, Barry S., Frederick S. Wilkinson, and William M. Marine. "Reducing Neonatal Mortality Rate with Nurse-Midwives." *American Journal of Obstetrics and Gynecology,* 109 (January 1971), 50-58.

Levy, Julius. "The Maternal and Infant Mortality in Midwifery Practice in Newark, New Jersey." *American Journal of Obstetrics and the Diseases of Women and Children,* 77 (1918), 41-53.

Levy, Walter E. "Our Midwife Problems." *Southern Medical Journal,* 24 (September 1931), 815-820.

Litzenberg, Jennings C. "A Child Is to Be Born." *Hygenia,* 4 (June 1926), 306-308.

Lobenstine, Ralph W. "The Influence of the Midwife Upon Infant and Maternal Morbidity and Mortality." *American Journal of Obstetrics and the Diseases of Women and Children,* 63 (1911), 876-880.

Lobenstine, Ralph W. "Saving Life by Prenatal Care." *Delineator,* 100 (July 1922), 17, 90-91.

Lubic, Ruth W. "Myths About Nurse-Midwifery." *American Journal of Nursing,* 74 (February 1974), 268-269.

Lynch, Frank W. "A Child Is to Be Born." *Hygenia,* 4 (May 1926), 253-255.

Mabbott, J. M. "The Regulation of Midwives in New York." *American Journal of Obstetrics and the Diseases of Women and Children,* 60 (1907), 516-527.

MacDonell, W. W. "Midwife Obstetrics." *Journal of the Florida Medical Association,* 6 (1919), 39-41.

Maeck, John Van S. "Obstetrician-Midwife Partnership in Obstetric Care." *Obstetrics and Gynecology,* 37 (February 1971), 314-319.

" 'Make Maternity Safe' is Mother's Day Slogan." *Hygenia,* 13 (May 1935), 471.

"Make Motherhood Safe for Mothers." *Hygenia,* 12 (May 1934), 403.

Mallon, Winifred. "Midwives in Relation to High Maternal Mortality." *Trained Nurse,* 82 (June 1929), 765-768.

Manley, T. H. "Women as Midwives." *Transactions of the New York State Medical Association,* 1 (1884), 370-375.

Marshall, E. A. "Interviews with Midwives." *Journal of the American Institute of Homeopathy,* 27 (February 1934), 109-111.

"Maternal Care and Infant Mortality." *Independent,* 67 (April 1909), 320-322.

"Maternal Death Rate Investigation, Children's Bureau." *New Republic,* 77 (December 1933), 87.

"Maternal Instinct Run Riot." *Good Housekeeping,* 52 (February 1911), 245-247.

"Maternity Death Rate: Mortality Survey Finds 65.8 Per Cent Preventable." *News-Week,* 2 (November 1933), 27.

McCord, James R. "The Education of Midwives." *American Journal of Obstetrics and Gynecology,* 21 (1931), 837-852.

McCoy, Samuel. "Ketchin' Babies: A Hundred Thousand Births that Need Safe Safeguarding." *Survey,* 54 (August 1925), 483-486.

McEvoy, J. P. "Our Streamlined Baby." *Reader's Digest,* 32 (May 1938), 15-18.

"Medieval Thinking About Childbirth." *Ladies' Home Journal,* 53 (October 1936), 4.

Meglen, Marie C., and Helen V. Burst. "Nurse-Midwives Make a Difference." *Nursing Outlook,* 22 (June 1974), 386-389.

Mengert, W. F. "Preparing for Baby." *Hygenia,* 17 (May 1939), 403-406.

"Midwife Supervision and Child Saving." *Survey,* 40 (August 1918), 566-567.

"Midwife Survey in Michigan." *Journal of the Michigan State Medical Society,* 24 (July 1925), 356.

Montell, Helen. "Charming Mothers-To-Be." *Ladies' Home Journal,* 46 (March 1929), 62.

Mooney, Belle S. "A Child Is to Be Born." *Hygenia,* 4 (October 1926), 581-582.

"Most Vital Statistics." *Commonweal,* 20 (June 1934), 115-116.

"Mothers and Children Last." *Survey,* 66 (April 1931), 93.

"Mothers Who Died." *Survey,* 69 (December 1933), 420.

Mumford, S. E. "Is Meddlesome Midwifery Bad?" *American Practitioner,* 16 (December 1877), 337-342.

Mustard, H. S. "Maternity and Child Hygiene." *Proceedings of the National Conference of Social Work* (1928), 203-213.

"Natal Narcotics." *Newsweek,* 11 (June 1938), 19.

"New Jersey's Midwives." *Survey,* 67 (October 1931), 92-93.

Newmayer, S. W. "The Status of Midwifery in Pennsylvania and a Study of the Midwives of Philadelphia." *Monthly Cyclopedia and Medical Bulletin,* 4 (1911), 712-719.

Nicholson, William R. "The Midwife Situation." *Transactions of the*

American Gynecology Society, 42 (1917), 623-631.

Noyes, Clara D. "The Training of Midwives in Relation to the Prevention of Infant Mortality." *American Journal of Obstetrics and the Diseases of Women and Children,* 66 (1912), 1051-1059.

Noyes, Frederick B. "A Child Is to Be Born." *Hygenia,* 4 (November 1926), 632.

"On the Opening of the Johns Hopkins Medical School to Women." *Century,* 19 (February 1891), 632-637.

Paalman, Russell J. "The Abundant Life: Presidential Address." *American Journal of Obstetrics and Gynecology,* 122 (May 1975), 139-143.

Paine, A. K. "The Midwife Problem." *Boston Medical and Surgical Journal,* 173 (November 1915), 759-764.

" 'Painless' Childbirth." *American Mercury,* 47 (June 1939), 220-224.

Peck, Harold A. "The Care of the Expectant Mother." *Hygenia,* 8 (August 1930), 720-722.

Peck, P. "Women Physicians and Their State Medical Societies." *Journal of the American Medical Women's Association,* 20 (April 1965), 351-353.

Peckham, C. H. "The Essentials of Adequate Maternal Care in Rural Areas." *The Child,* 4 (November 1939), 119-124.

Penman, W. R. "The Public Practice of Midwifery in Philadelphia." *Transactions and Studies of the College of Physicians of Philadelphia,* 37 (October 1969), 124-132.

Plecker, W. A. "The First Move Toward Midwife Control in Virginia." *Virginia Medical Monthly,* 45 (April 1918), 12-13.

Plecker, W. A. "The Midwife in Virginia." *Virginia Medical Semi-Monthly,* 18 (January 1914), 474-477.

Plecker, W. A. "The Midwife Problem in Virginia." *Virginia Medical Semi-Monthly,* 19 (December 1914), 456-458.

Plecker, W. A. "Virginia Makes Efforts to Solve Midwife Problem." *Nation's Health,* 7 (December 1925), 809-811.

Poole, E. "Nurse on Horseback: Frontier Nursing Service." *Good Housekeeping,* 94 (June 1932), 38-39, 203-210.

Pringle, Henry F. "What Do the Women of America Think About Medicine?" *Ladies' Home Journal,* 55 (September 1938), 14-15, 42-43.

Pryor, J. H. "The Status of the Midwife in Buffalo." *New York Medical Journal,* 11 (August 1884), 129-132.

"Public Demands and the Medical Education of Women." *Nation,* 50 (March 1890), 237-238.

Purrington, W. A. "The Midwifery Question." *Medical Record,* 53 (February 1898), 286-287.

Putnam, W. L. "Prenatal Care." *Proceedings of the National Conference of Charities and Corrections* (1911), 349-354.

Putnam, W. L. "Pre-Natal Care of the Next Generation." *Survey,* 29 (January 1913), 437-439.

"Rebirth of the Midwife." *Life,* 71 (November 1971), 50-55.

Reese, D. Meredith. "Report on Infant Mortality in Large Cities, the Sources of Its Increase, and Means for Its Diminution." *Transactions of the American Medical Association,* 10 (1857), 93-107.

"Registration of Midwives." *Medical Record,* 48 (September 1895), 449-450.

Reid, Ada Chree. "Those Were the Days." *Journal of the American Medical Women's Association,* 2 (1956), 140-141.

"Relief of Pain in Childbirth." *Hygenia,* 14 (June 1936), 558.

Richardson, Anna S. "Safeguarding American Motherhood." *McClure's,* 45 (July 1915), 35.

Richardson, Anna S. "Safety First for Mother." *McClure's,* 45 (May 1915), 24, 97-100.

Rivington, Ann. "Motherhood—Third Class." *American Mercury,* 31 (February 1934), 160-165.

Robinson, Charles A. "Extern: How the Babies of the Slums Are Brought into the World." *Century,* 115 (March 1928), 551-560.

"Role of the Nurse-Midwife." *American Journal of Obstetrics and Gynecology,* 124 (March 1976), 666-667.

Ross, R. A. "Granny Grandiosity." *Southern Medicine and Surgery,* 96 (February 1934), 57-59.

Rothman, Barbara Katz. "Woman's Body/Woman's Mind: In Which a Sensible Woman Persuades Her Doctor, Her Family, and Her Friends to Help Her Give Birth at Home." *Ms.,* 5 (December 1976), 25-32.

Royer, B. F. "Midwives in Pennsylvania." *Pennsylvania Medical Journal,* 16 (January 1913), 289-294.

Sargent, C. A. "Midwifery in Delaware." *Delaware State Medical Journal,* 5 (August 1933), 176-177.

Savage, Clara S. "It Can Happen Here: Reduction in Maternity Deaths." *Parents' Magazine,* 12 (May 1937), 17.

Schuler, L. A. "They Need Not Have Died." *Ladies' Home Journal,* 51 (February 1934), 22.

Shaver, Elizabeth. "Infant Mortality and the Midwife Problem." *Louisville (Kentucky) Monthly Journal of Medicine and Surgery,* 19 (June 1912), 24-29.

Slemons, Josiah Morris. "Care of Prospective Mothers." *Outlook,* 16 (May 1917), 110-111.

Slome, C. "Effectiveness of Certified Nurse-Midwives." *American Journal of Obstetrics and Gynecology,* 124 (January 1976), 177-182.

Smith, Helena H. "Back to the Midwife?" *New Republic,* 79 (July 1934),
   207.

Smith, Helena H. "The Case for Anesthesia." *Delineator,* 125 (September
   1934), 30, 50-51.

Smith, W. S. "Careless and Unscientific Midwifery, with Special Reference
   to Some Features of the Work of Midwives." *Maryland Medical Journal,*
   33 (1895-1896), 146-149.

Solenberger, Edith R. "Nurses on Horseback, Frontier Nursing Service."
   Hygenia, 9 (July 1931), 633-638.

Southmyard, Leotha B. "Motherhood-Third Class—A Reply." *American
   Mercury,* 31 (April 1934), 509-510.

Spencer, Herbert R. "The Renaissance of Midwifery." *Transactions of the
   Medical Society of London,* 48 (1925), 71-105.

Steele, Guy. "The Midwife Problem and Its Legal Control." *Maryland
   Medical Journal,* 48 (January 1905), 1-6.

Stewart, Jane. "Is the Mother Ready for the Baby?" *Ladies' Home Journal,*
   30 (February 1913), 76.

Stone, Ellen A. "The Midwives of Rhode Island." *Providence Medical
   Journal,* 13 (1912), 57-60.

Streshinsky, Shirley. "Are You Safer with a Midwife?" *Ms.,* 2 (October
   1973), 24-27.

Studdiford, W. E. "Attempts at Regulation of Midwife Practice." *American
   Journal of Obstetrics and the Diseases of Women and Children,* 63
   (1911), 898-901.

Teller, Charlotte. "The Neglected Psychology of the 'Twilight Sleep.'" *Good
   Housekeeping,* 61 (July 1915), 17-24.

Terry, Charles E. "Midwife Menace." *Delineator,* 91 (October 1917), 15-16.

Terry, Charles E. "The Mother, the Midwife and the Law." *Delineator,*
   92 (February 1916), 12-13.

Terry, Charles E. "Save the Seventh Baby." *Delineator,* 92 (October 1917),
   15-16, 48, 50.

"This Motherhood Bunk." *American Mercury,* 45 (November 1938), 287-289.

Thomas, G. Morton. "Removal of the Ovaries as a Cure for Insanity."
   American Journal of Insanity, 49 (1892-1893), 397-401.

Thomas, Margaret. "Wanted: Someone to Care for 250,000 Women."
   Briefs, 7 (May 1942), 51.

Thompson, O. R. "Midwife Problem." *Journal of the Medical Association
   of Georgia,* 16 (April 1927), 135-139.

Thoms, Herbert. "A Wider Outlook in Obstetrics." *American Journal of
   Obstetrics and Gynecology,* 76 (December 1956), 1305-1308.

Todd, Constance L. "Easier Motherhood." *Ladies' Home Journal*, 47 (March 1930), 9, 204, 207, 209.

Tracy, Marguerite, and Constance Leupp. "Painless Childbirth." *McClure's*, 43 (June 1914), 37-51.

Tuttle, Margaret M. "Maternity and the Woman Intellectual." *Collier's*, 44 (January 1910), 18-19.

Underwood, Felix J. "The Development of Midwifery in Mississippi." *Southern Medical Journal*, 19 (September 1926), 683-687.

Van Blarcom, Carolyn C. "Awaiting the First Baby." *Delineator*, 97 (October 1920), 40.

Van Blarcom, Carolyn C. "Has the Nursing Profession a Responsibility in Connection Midwives?" *British Journal of Nursing*, 74 (September 1926), 212-214.

Van Blarcom, Carolyn C. "A Possible Solution of the Midwife Problem." *Proceedings of the National Conference of Charities and Correction* (1910), 350-356.

Van Blarcom, Carolyn C. "Prenatal Days, and Cheerful, Too." *Delineator*, 97 (September 1920), 34, 54.

Van Blarcom, Carolyn C. "Rat Pie: Among the Black Midwives of the South." *Harper's*, 160 (February 1930), 322-332.

Van Ingen, Philip. "Education of Mothers and the Saving of Babies." *Proceedings of the Academy of Political Science*, 2 (July 1912), 669-672.

Van Peyma, P. W. "The Midwife." *Buffalo Medical Journal*, 66 (1910-1911), 477-486.

Vaughn, Victor C. "Infantile Mortality: Its Causation and Its Reduction." *Journal of the American Medical Association*, 14 (February 1890), 181-185.

Von Ramdohr, C. A. "Midwifery and Midwife." *Medical Record*, 3 (December 1897), 882-883.

Wadsworth, L. C. "The Midwife and Midwifery." *American Practitioner and News*, 26 (1898), 209-212.

Wallace, Helen M., Curtis L. Mendelson, Leona Baumgartner, and Ruth Rothmayer. "The Practice of Midwives in New York City." *New York State Journal of Medicine*, 48 (January 1948), 67-71.

Watson, B. P. "Can Our Methods of Obstetric Practice be Improved?" *Bulletin of the New York Academy of Medicine*, 6 (October 1930), 647-663.

Welshimer, Helen. "Two Out of Three Can Be Saved." *Good Housekeeping*, 102 (June 1936), 60-61.

Welz, Walter E. "Michigan's Midwife Problem." *Journal of the Michigan State Medical Society*, 21 (December 1912), 788-793.

"We Must All Care." *Ladies' Home Journal*, 53 (December 1936), 4.

"When Mothers Die It's News." *Nation*, 138 (January 1934), 118.

Whitridge, J., and E. Davens. "Are Public Health Maternity Programs Effective and Necessary?" *American Journal of Public Health*, 42 (May 1952), 508-515.

Wile, Ira S. "Immigration and Midwife Problems." *Boston Medical and Surgical Journal*, 167 (1912), 113-115.

Wile, Ira S. "Immigration and the Midwife Problem." *Bulletin of the American Academy of Medicine*, 4 (1913), 197-202.

Wile, Ira S. "Schools for Midwives." *Medical Record*, 81 (March 1912), 517-518.

Wiley, Harvey W. "Diet for the Expectant Mother." *Good Housekeeping*, 64 (April 1917), 53-54.

Wiley, Harvey W. "Getting Ready for Baby." *Good Housekeeping*, 74 (April 1922), 59.

Williams, J. W. "The Plan as Adopted by Beaufort County for the Control of Midwifery." *New Albany Medical Herald*, 35 (1926), 134-137.

Williams, L. R. "Position of the New York State Department of Health Relative to Control of Midwives." *New York State Journal of Medicine*, 15 (August 1915), 296-301.

Wilson, Robert J. "Health Care for Women: Present Deficiencies and Future Needs." *Obstetrics and Gynecology*, 36 (August 1970), 178-185.

"Women in Medicine." *Saturday Evening Post*, 200 (January 1928), 22.

Woods, Hiram. "Professional Significance of the Midwife and Optometry Bills Passed by the Recent Legislature of Maryland." *Maryland Medical Journal*, 53 (June 1910), 189-196.

Worden, H. "She Nurses Her Patients for a Dollar a Year." *American Magazine*, 112 (December 1931), 69-70, 108.

World Health Organization. "Expert Committee on Midwifery Training, First Report." August 2-7, 1954. *World Health Organization Technical Report Series*, 93 (1955), 3-21.

Young, J. Van D. "The Midwife Problem in the State of New York." *New York State Journal of Medicine*, 15 (1915), 291-296.

Zabriskie, Louise. "Expectant Mothers: Preparing for the Baby's Birth." *Parents' Magazine*, 6 (March 1931), 70-71.

Miscellaneous

Atlanta Constitution. October 31, 1975.

Atlanta Constitution. September 16, 1974.

New York Sun. June 8, 1933.

New York Times. March 27, 1976.

Providence Evening Bulletin. December 27, 1976.

Supplement, United States Daily. April 6, 1931.
Interview with Adele Alexandre, participant at the First International Conference of Practicing Midwives. Providence, R.I., January 20, 1977.

Müller, Susanna, 1756-1785. An Old German Midwife's Record. Edited by M. D. Learned and C. F. Bride, [n.p., n.d.]. Located at the Library of the College of Physicians of Philadelphia.

Program Notes, Rhode Island Women's Health Conference, Providence, R.I., March 27, 1976.

Ventre, Fran. "Proposal for Education of Certified Midwives." Mimeographed. Washington, D.C.: HOME, 1976.

United States Government Publications
—Children's Bureau

Allen, Nila F. *Infant Mortality: Results of a Field Study in Saginaw, Michigan. Based on Births in One Year.* United States Department of Labor, Children's Bureau Publication, No. 52. Washington, D.C.: Government Printing Office, 1919.

Baby-Saving Campaigns: A Preliminary Report on What American Cities Are Doing to Prevent Infant Mortality. United States Department of Labor, Children's Bureau Publication, No. 3. Washington, D.C.: Government Printing Office, 1913.

Births, Infant Mortality, Maternal Mortality, 1940. United States Department of Labor, Children's Bureau Publication, No. 288. Washington, D.C.: Government Printing Office, 1943.

Bradbury, Dorothy E. *Five Decades of Action for Children: A History of the Children's Bureau.* United States Department of Health, Education and Welfare, Children's Bureau Publication, No. 358. Washington, D.C.: Government Printing Office, 1962.

Child Care and Child Welfare. United States Department of Labor, Children's Bureau Publication, No. 90. Washington, D.C.: Government Printing Office, 1921.

Dart, Helen M. *Maternity and Child Care in Selected Rural Areas in Mississippi.* United States Department of Labor, Children's Bureau Publication, No. 88. Washington, D.C.: Government Printing Office, 1921.

Dempsey, Mary V. *Infant Mortality: Results of a Field Study in Brockton, Massachusetts. Based on Births in One Year.* United States Department of Labor, Children's Bureau Publication, No. 37. Washington, D.C.: Government Printing Office, 1919.

Duke, Emma. *Infant Mortality: Results of a Field Study in Johnstown, Pennsylvania. Based on Births in One Calendar Year.* United States Department of Labor, Children's Bureau Publication, No. 9. Washington, D.C.: Government Printing Office, 1915.

Duncan, Beatrice Sheets, and Emma Duke. *Infant Mortality: Results of a Field Study in Manchester, New Hampshire. Based on Births in One Year.* United States Department of Labor, Children's Bureau Publication, No. 20. Washington, D.C.: Government Printing Office, 1917.

Haley, Theresa S. *Infant Mortality: Results of a Field Study in Akron, Ohio. Based on Births in One Year.* United States Department of Labor, Children's Bureau Publication, No. 72. Washington, D.C.: Government Printing Office, 1920.

Hughes, Elizabeth. *Infant Mortality: Results of a Field Study in Gary, Indiana. Based on Births in One Year.* United States Department of Labor, Children's Bureau Publication, No. 112. Washington, D.C.: Government Printing Office, 1923.

Hunt, Eleanor P. *Recent Demographic Trends and Their Effects on Maternal and Child Health Needs and Services.* United States Department of Health, Education and Welfare, Children's Bureau Publication. Washington, D.C.: Government Printing Office, 1966.

Hunter, Estelle B. *Infant Mortality: Results of a Field Study in Waterbury, Connecticut. Based on Births in One Year.* United States Department of Labor, Children's Bureau Publication, No. 29. Washington, D.C.: Government Printing Office, 1918.

Infant Mortality, Montclair, New Jersey: A Study of Infant Mortality in a Suburban Community. United States Department of Labor, Children's Bureau Publication, No. 11. Washington, D.C.: Government Printing Office, 1915.

Jones, Anita M. *Manual for Teaching Midwives.* United States Department of Labor, Children's Bureau Publication, No. 260. Washington, D.C.: Government Printing Office, 1941.

Maternal Deaths: A Brief Report of a Study Made in Fifteen States. United States Department of Labor, Children's Bureau Publication, No. 221. Washington, D.C.: Government Printing Office, 1933.

Maternal Mortality in Fifteen States. United States Department of Labor, Children's Bureau Publication, No. 223. Washington, D.C.: Government Printing Office, 1934.

Meigs, Grace L. *Maternal Mortality From All Conditions Connected With Childbirth in the United States and Certain Other Countries.* United

States Department of Labor, Children's Bureau Publication, No. 19. Washington, D.C.: Government Printing Office, 1917.

Minimum Standards for Child Welfare. United States Department of Labor, Children's Bureau Publication, No. 62. Washington, D.C.: Government Printing Office, 1919.

Moore, Elizabeth. *Maternity and Infant Care in a Rural County in Kansas.* United States Department of Labor, Children's Bureau Publication, No. 26. Washington, D.C.: Government Printing Office, 1917.

Paradise, Viola I. *Maternity Care and the Welfare of Young Children in a Homesteading County in Montana.* United States Department of Labor, Children's Bureau Publication, No. 34. Washington, D.C.: Government Printing Office, 1919.

Proceedings of the Third Annual Conference of State Directors in Charge of the Local Administration of the Maternity and Infancy Act. United States Department of Labor, Children's Bureau Publication, No. 157. Washington, D.C.: Government Printing Office, 1926.

Rochester, Anna. *Infant Mortality: Results of a Field Study in Baltimore, Maryland. Based on Births in One Year.* United States Department of Labor, Children's Bureau Publication, No. 119. Washington, D.C.: Government Printing Office, 1923.

Save the Youngest: Seven Charts on Maternal and Infant Mortality with Explanatory Comment. United States Department of Labor, Children's Bureau Publication, No. 61. Washington, D.C.: Government Printing Office, [1919].

Sherbon, Florence Brown, and Elizabeth Moore. *Maternity and Infant Care in Two Rural Counties in Wisconsin.* United States Department of Labor, Children's Bureau Publication, No. 46. Washington, D.C.: Government Printing Office, 1919.

Standards of Child Welfare: A Report of the Children's Bureau Conferences. United States Department of Labor, Children's Bureau Publication, No. 60. Washington, D.C.: Government Printing Office, 1919.

Standards of Prenatal Care: An Outline for the Use of Physicians. United States Department of Labor, Children's Bureau Publication, No. 153. Washington, D.C.: Government Printing Office, 1925.

Steele, Glenn. *Maternity and Infant Care in a Mountain County in Georgia.* United States Department of Labor, Children's Bureau Publication, No. 120. Washington, D.C.: Government Printing Office, 1923.

Tandy, Elizabeth. *Comparability of Maternal Mortality Rates in the United States and Certain Foreign Countries.* United States Department of Labor, Children's Bureau Publication, No. 229. Washington, D.C.: Government Printing Office, 1935.

Tandy, Elizabeth. *Infant and Maternal Mortality Among Negroes.* United States Department of Labor, Children's Bureau Publication, No. 243. Washington, D.C.: Government Printing Office, 1937.

Thomas, Margaret W. *The Practice of Nurse-Midwifery in the United States.* United States Department of Health, Education and Welfare, Children's Bureau Publication, No. 436. Washington, D.C.: Government Printing Office, 1965.

Whitney, Jessamine S. *Infant Mortality: Results of a Field Study in New Bedford, Massachusetts. Based on Births in One Year.* United States Department of Labor, Children's Bureau Publication, No. 68. Washington, D.C.: Government Printing Office, 1920.

Woodbury, Robert M. *Maternal Mortality: The Risk of Death in Childbirth and From All Diseases Caused by Pregnancy and Confinement.* United States Department of Labor, Children's Bureau Publication, No. 158. Washington, D.C.: Government Printing Office, 1926.

United States Government Publications
—Miscellaneous

Campbell, Janet M. "Training of Midwives." *Public Health Reports,* 39 (February 1924), 341-348.

Lee, Florence Ellen, and Jay H. Glasser. "Role of Lay Midwifery in Maternity Care in a Large Metropolitan Area." *Public Health Reports,* 89 (November-December 1974), 537-544.

Practice of Medicine and Midwifery in the District of Columbia. Hearing before a subcommittee, 69th Congress, 2d session on S. 441, to regulate the practice of medicine and midwifery in the District of Columbia and to punish persons violating provisions thereof. January 5, 1927.

Rude, Anna E. *The Sheppard-Towner Act in Relation to Public Health.* Washington, D.C., 1922.

United States Bureau of the Census. *Historical Statistics of the United States, Colonial Times to 1957.* Washington, D.C., 1960.

United States Bureau of the Census. *Statistical Abstract of the United States: 1973.* 94th edition. Washington, D.C., 1973.

United States Bureau of the Census. *Statistical Abstract of the United States: 1975.* 96th edition. Washington, D.C., 1975.

United States Bureau of the Census. *Vital Statistics of the United States.* 1937-1970 annual volumes. Washington, D.C.

Williams, R. C. *The United States Public Health Service, 1789-1950.* Washington, D.C.: United States Public Health Service, 1951.

State and Local Publications

ALABAMA

Laws Regulating the Practice of Midwifery in Alabama. Alabama State Board of Health, 1928.

Marriner, Jessie L. *Midwifery in Alabama.* Alabama State Board of Health, [1925].

ARIZONA

Midwife Safety Rules. Arizona State Board of Health, 1924.

CONNECTICUT

Bulletin. Connecticut State Department of Health. 1 (1887)-44 (1930).

Report. Connecticut State Department of Health, 1879-1930.

State Statutes Concerning the Practice of Midwifery. Connecticut State Department of Health, [1923].

GEORGIA

All My Babies. Georgia Department of Public Health, Miscellaneous Files, Box 1. Included in Box 1 is information pertaining to the circumstances which led to the production of the 1953 film, *All My Babies.* The film was produced by the Georgia Department of Public Health during the early 1950s. It was shot in Georgia and features a black, certified lay midwife, her patients and their families, and the doctors and nurses who supervised the lay midwife program. A copy of this unique film is located at the Georgia State Department of Archives and History, Atlanta, Georgia.

Bulletin. Georgia State Board of Health. 1911, 1913, 1914, 1917, 1918, 1919.

"Georgia Midwife Plan." Mimeographed. Georgia Department of Public Health, Miscellaneous Files, Box 1 [193?].

Lessons for Midwives. Georgia State Board of Health, Miscellaneous Files, Box 1 [1922].

Maternal Health and Family Planning. Georgia Department of Public Health, Miscellaneous File, Boxes 1, 2, and 3.

Midwife Manual. Georgia Department of Public Health, Miscellaneous Files, Box 1 [April 3, 1937].

Minutes. Georgia State Board of Health, 1903-1930.

Regulations Governing the Practice of Midwifery, January 28, 1925. Georgia State Board of Health, Miscellaneous Files, Box 1.

Report. Georgia State Board of Health, 1875-1876, 1904-1908, 1919-1932.

Resolution Adopted by the Medical Association of Georgia Concerning the Practice of Midwifery in Georgia, May 9, 1924. Georgia Department of Public Health, Miscellaneous Files, Box 1.

Savannah Board of Sanitary Commissions. *Memo Concerning the Regulation of Midwives, 1922.* Georgia Department of Public Health, Miscellaneous Files, Box 1.

Winchester, M. E. *Official Bulletin on A Brief History of Public Health Work in Georgia.* Atlanta: Georgia State Board of Health, 1927.

ILLINOIS

Report of the Health Insurance Commission of the State of Illinois. State of Illinois, 1919.

"Requirements for Midwives." *Monthly Bulletin,* Illinois State Board of Health, 6 (October 1910), 393-409.

LOUISIANA

Lange, Deola. "The Midwife at the Present." *Quarterly Bulletin.* Louisiana Department of Health, 40 (September 1949), 10-18.

Ziegler, Azelie. "The Midwife of the Past." *Quarterly Bulletin.* Louisiana Department of Health, 40 (September 1949), 5-10.

MAINE

Acts and Resolves of the Legislature of the State of Maine. 67th Legislature (1895); 75th Legislature (1911).

Baby, The. Maine State Department of Health, [1939].

Bulletin. Maine State Department of Health, 1905-1922.

Expectant Mother, The. Maine State Department of Health, [1939].

Manual for Public Health Nurses. Maine State Bureau of Health, 1946.

Report. Maine State Board of Health, 1885-1917.

MARYLAND

An Act to Provide for the Registration and Licensing of Midwives in the State of Maryland. 1912.

MASSACHUSETTS

Acts and Resolves Passed by the Legislature of Massachusetts. 1894.

Annual Report. Massachusetts Department of Public Health, 1900-1923.

Commonhealth. Massachusetts Department of Public Health, 7 (1920)-17 (1930).

Commonwealth v. *Hanna Porn. Massachusetts Reports.* 195, 196 (1907).

Documents. House of Representatives, Commonwealth of Massachusetts, 1913-1914.

Journal of the House of Representatives. Commonwealth of Massachusetts, 1913.

Monthly Bulletin. Massachusetts State Board of Health, 1 (1906)-9 (1914).

Public Health Bulletin. Massachusetts Department of Health, 1 (1914)-6 (1919).

Revised Laws of the Commonwealth of Massachusetts. 1901.

Weekly Bulletin. Massachusetts State Board of Health, 1 (1883)-23 (1905).

MINNESOTA

Correspondence Study Course in the Hygiene of Maternity and Infancy. Minnesota State Department of Health, 1925-1928.

MISSISSIPPI

Manual for Midwives. Mississippi State Board of Health, 1927, 1933, 1962.

Miscellaneous Mimeographed Information Including Letters of Notification of Midwife Club Meetings and Outline for Nurses Giving Instructions to Midwives. Mississippi State Board of Health, 1927-1928.

Report. Board of Health of Mississippi, 1919-1923.

Underwood, Felix J. *Public Health and Medical Licensure in the State of Mississippi, 1798-1937.* Jackson: Mississippi State Board of Health, 1938.

NEW JERSEY

Annual Report. New Jersey State Department of Health, 1926, 1928.

Progressive Midwife. New Jersey State Department of Health, 1927-1932.

NEW MEXICO

Regulations Governing the Practice of Midwifery, November 20, 1922. New Mexico Bureau of Public Health.

NEW YORK CITY

Legal Duties of Physicians, Midwives, Undertakers and Cemetery Keepers. New York City Department of Health, 1910.

"Maternal Mortality in New York City." *Weekly Bulletin,* Department of Health, City of New York, 10 (May 1921), 169-171.

"Memorandum Re: Control and Practice of Midwifery in New York City." Mimeographed. New York City Bureau of Municipal Research, 1915.

Regulations Governing the Practice of Midwifery in the City of New York. New York City Department of Health, 1918.

"Supervision of Midwives in New York City." *Weekly Bulletin*, Department of Health, City of New York, 10 (May 1921), 153-157.

Thomas, Lee W. "The Supervision of Midwives in New York City." *Monthly Bulletin*, Department of Health, City of New York, 9 (May 1919), 117-120.

NEW YORK STATE

An Act to Amend the Public Health Law, in Relation to the Practice of Midwifery, January 6, 1913. New York State Legislature Assembly.

De Porte, Joseph V. *Maternal Mortality and Stillbirths in New York State: 1915-1925.* Albany: New York State Department of Health, 1928.

NORTH CAROLINA

Promotion of the Welfare and Hygiene of Maternity and Infancy. North Carolina State Board of Health, [n.d.].

PENNSYLVANIA

Pennsylvania Baby Book. Pennsylvania Department of Health, 1922.

RHODE ISLAND

Biennial Report. Rhode Island Public Health Commission, 1929-1930.

Bulletin. Rhode Island State Board of Health, 1888-1918.

Report. Rhode Island State Board of Health, 1878-1928.

SOUTH CAROLINA

Regulations Governing Midwives. South Carolina State Board of Health, 1920.

TEXAS

"Report of the Midwife Survey in Texas." Mimeographed. Texas State Board of Health, 1924.

VIRGINIA

Midwife Instruction: A Series of Lectures Prepared for Virginia Nurses. Virginia State Board of Health, 1924.

SECONDARY SOURCES

Books and Pamphlets

Alsop, Gulielma Fell. *History of the Women's Medical College, Philadelphia, Pennsylvania, 1850-1950.* Philadelphia: J. B. Lippincott, 1950.

Aveling, J. H. *English Midwives, Their History and Prospects.* Reprint of 1872 edition. London: Elliot, Ltd., 1967.

Barker-Benfield, G. J. *The Horrors of the Half-Known Life: Male Attitudes Toward Women and Sexuality in Nineteenth-Century America.* New York: Harper & Row, Publishers, 1976.

Beard, Mary. *The Nurse in Public Health.* New York: Harper & Brothers, Publishers, 1929.

Boston Women's Health Collective. *Our Bodies, Ourselves: A Book By and For Women.* New York: Simon & Schuster, 1976.

Bremner, Robert H. *From the Depths: The Discovery of Poverty in the United States.* New York: New York University Press, 1956.

Brennan, Barbara, and Joan Rattner Heilman. *The Complete Book of Midwifery.* New York: E. P. Dutton & Company, Inc., 1977.

Brown, Harriet Conner. *Grandmother Brown's Hundred Years, 1827-1927.* Boston: Little, Brown & Company, 1929.

Burrow, James G. *AMA: Voice of American Medicine.* Baltimore: Johns Hopkins University Press, 1963.

Campbell, Marie. *Folks Do Get Born.* New York: Rinehart & Company, 1946.

Cianfrani, Theodore. *A Short History of Obstetrics and Gynecology.* Springfield, Ill.: C. C. Thomas, 1960.

Corner, Betsy E. *William Shippen, Jr., Pioneer in American Medical Education.* Philadelphia: American Philosophical Society, 1951.

Corwin, E. H. L. *The American Hospital.* New York: The Commonwealth Fund, 1946.

Cowen, David L. *Medicine and Health in New Jersey: A History.* Vol. XVI of *The New Jersey Historical Society Series,* eds. Richard M. Huber and Wheaton J. Lane. Princeton, N.J.: D. Van Nostrand Company, Inc., 1964.

Crawford, Susan. *Digest of Official Actions: American Medical Association, 1846-1958.* [Chicago]: American Medical Association, 1959.

Cutter, Irving S., and Henry R. Viets. *A Short History of Midwifery.* Philadelphia: W. B. Saunders, 1964.

Derbyshire, R. C. *Medical Licensure and Discipline in the United States.* Baltimore: Johns Hopkins University Press, 1969.

Dexter, Elizabeth A. *Career Women of America: 1776-1840.* Francetown, N.H.: M. Jones, 1950.

Dexter, Elizabeth A. *Colonial Women of Affairs: Women in Business and Professions in America before 1776.* Boston: Houghton & Mifflin, 1931.

Dolan, Josephine A., ed. *History of Nursing.* 12th edition. Philadelphia: W. B. Saunders, 1968.

Duffy, John. *A History of Public Health in New York City, 1866-1966.* New York: Russell Sage Foundation, 1974.

Ehrenreich, Barbara, and Deidre English. *Complaints and Disorders: The Sexual Politics of Sickness.* New York: The Feminist Press, 1973.

Ehrenreich, Barbara, and Deidre English. *Witches, Midwives, and Nurses: A History of Women Healers.* Oyster Bay, N.Y.: Glass Mountain Pamphlets, [1973].

Ernst, Christopher Meyer. *Infant Mortality in New York City: A Study of the Results Accomplished by Infant-Life Saving Agencies, 1885-1920.* New York: The Rockefeller Foundation, 1921.

Findley, Palmer. *Priests of Lucina: The Story of Obstetrics.* Boston: Little, Brown and Company, 1939.

Fishbein, Morris. *A History of the American Medical Association, 1847-1947.* Philadelphia: W. B. Saunders, 1947.

Flexner, J. T. *Doctors on Horseback: Pioneers of American Medicine.* New York: Garden City Publishing Company, 1939.

Frank, Sister Ch. Marie. *Foundations of Nursing.* 2nd edition. Philadelphia: W.B. Saunders, 1959.

Galishoff, Stuart. *Safeguarding the Public Health: Newark, 1895-1918.* Westport, Conn.: Greenwood Press, 1975.

Garceau, Oliver. *The Political Life of the American Medical Association.* Cambridge, Mass.: Harvard University Press, 1941.

Garrison, Fielding H. *An Introduction to the History of Medicine.* 4th edition. Philadelphia: W. B. Saunders, 1929.

Goldmark, Josephine. *Impatient Crusader: Florence Kelley's Life Story.* Urbana, Ill.: University of Illinois Press, 1953.

Goodnow, Minnie. *Nursing History.* 7th edition. Philadelphia: W. B. Saunders, 1942.

Gordon, Linda. *Woman's Body, Woman's Right: A Social History of Birth Control in America.* New York: Grossman Publishers, 1976.

Grabill, Wilson H., Clyde V. Kiser, and Pascal K. Whelpton. *The Fertility of American Women.* New York: John Wiley & Sons, 1958.

Graham, Harvey. *Eternal Eve: The Mysteries of Birth and the Customs That Surround It.* London: Hutchinson & Company, 1960.

Haggard, Howard W. *Devils, Drugs, and Doctors: The Story of the Science of Healing from Medicine-Man to Doctor.* New York: Harper & Brothers, Publishers, 1929.

Haire, Doris B. *The Cultural Warping of Childbirth.* Seattle, Wash.: International Childbirth Education Association, 1972.

Hall, David D., ed. *The Antinomian Controversy, 1636-1638.* Middletown, Conn.: Wesleyan University Press, 1968.

Haller, Mark H. *Eugenics: Hereditarian Attitudes in American Thought.*

New Brunswick, N.J.: Rutgers University Press, 1963.

Harris, Seale. *Woman's Surgeon: The Life Story of J. Marion Sims.* New York: Macmillan Company, 1950.

Health Policy Advisory Committee. *The American Health Empire: Power, Profits, and Politics.* New York: Random House, 1970.

Henry, Frederick P., ed. *Founders Week Memorial Volume.* Philadelphia: City of Philadelphia, 1909.

Higham, John. *Strangers in the Land: Patterns of American Nativism, 1860-1925.* New York: Atheneum, 1970.

Himes, Norman E. *Medical History of Contraception.* Baltimore: Williams & Wilkins Company, 1936.

Hume, Ruth Fox. *Great Women of Medicine.* New York: Random House, 1964.

Hurd-Mead, Kate Campbell. *A History of Women in Medicine.* Haddam, Conn.: Haddam Press, 1938.

Hurd-Mead, Kate Campbell. *Medical Women of America.* New York: Froben Press, 1933.

Kett, Joseph. *The Formation of the American Medical Profession, 1780-1860.* New Haven, Conn.: Yale University Press, 1968.

Kiser, C. V., W. H. Grabill, and A. A. Campbell. *Trends and Variations in Fertility in the United States.* Cambridge, Mass.: Harvard University Press, 1968.

Laufe, Leonard. *Obstetric Forceps.* New York: Harper & Row, Publishers, 1968.

Lemons, J. Stanley. *The Woman Citizen: Social Feminism in the 1920's.* Urbana, Ill.: University of Illinois, 1973.

Lopate, Carol. *Women in Medicine.* Baltimore: Johns Hopkins University Press, 1968.

Lovejoy, Esther P. *Women Doctors of the World.* New York: Macmillan Company, 1957.

Marshall, Clara. *The Woman's Medical College of Pennsylvania.* Philadelphia: P. Blakiston, Son & Company, 1897.

McCleary, G. F. *The Early History of the Infant Welfare Movement.* London: H. K. Lewis & Company, 1933.

Morris, Richard B., ed. *Encyclopedia of American History.* New York: Harper & Row, Publishers, 1965.

Nash, Charles E. *The History of Augusta: First Settlements and Early Days as A Town, Including the Diary of Mrs. Martha Moore Ballard.* Augusta, Me.: Charles E. Nash & Sons, 1905.

New York Infirmary. *The New York Infirmary: A Century of Devoted Service.* New York: New York Infirmary, 1954.

Okun, Bernard. *Trends in Birth Rates in the United States Since 1870.*

Baltimore: Johns Hopkins University Press, 1958.

Packard, Francis R. *History of Medicine in the United States.* 2 vols. New York: Paul B. Hoeber, 1931.

Radcliffe, Walter. *Milestones in Midwifery.* Bristol, England: John Wright & Sons, Ltd., 1967.

Ravenel, Mazych, ed. *A Half Century of Public Health: Jubilee Historical Volume of the American Public Health Association.* New York: American Public Health Association, 1921.

Rayack, Elton. *Professional Power and American Medicine.* Cleveland: The World Publishing Company, 1967.

Ricci, James V. *The Development of Gynecological Surgery and Instruments.* Philadelphia: P. Blakiston, Son & Company, 1949.

Roberts, Mary M. *American Nursing: History and Interpretation.* New York: Macmillan Company, 1954.

Rockefeller Foundation. *Laws Governing the Practice of Midwifery (1904-1930).* New York: Rockefeller Foundation, 1931.

Ronzy, Abraham J. *Childbirth, Yesterday and Today.* New York: Emerson Books, Inc., 1937.

Rosen, George. *A History of Public Health.* New York: MD Publications, Inc., 1958.

Rosenberg, Charles E. *The Cholera Years: The United States in 1832, 1849, and 1866.* Chicago: University of Chicago Press, 1962.

Ross, Ishbel. *Child of Destiny: The Life Story of the First Woman Doctor.* New York: Harper & Brothers, Publishers, 1949.

Rothstein, William G. *American Physicians in the Nineteenth Century: From Sects to Science.* Baltimore: Johns Hopkins University Press, 1972.

Ruzek, Sheryl K. *Women and Health Care: A Bibliography with Selected Annotation.* Evanston, Ill.: The Program on Women, Northwestern University, 1976.

Shafer, Henry B. *The American Medical Profession, 1783-1850.* New York: Columbia University Press, 1936.

Shapiro, Sam, Edward R. Schlesinger, and Robert E. L. Nesbitt, Jr. *Infant, Perinatal, Maternal, and Childhood Mortality in the United States.* Cambridge, Mass.: Harvard University Press, 1968.

Shoemaker, M. Theopane. *History of Nurse-Midwifery in the United States.* Washington, D.C.: Catholic University Press, 1947.

Shryock, Richard H. *The Development of Modern Medicine: An Interpretation of the Social and Scientific Factors Involved.* New York: Alfred A. Knopf, 1947.

Shryock, Richard H. *The History of Nursing: An Interpretation of the*

Social and Medical Factors Involved. Philadelphia: W. B. Saunders, 1959.

Shryock, Richard H. *Medical Licensing in America, 1650-1965.* Baltimore: Johns Hopkins University Press, 1967.

Shryock, Richard H. *Medicine and Society in America, 1660-1860.* New York: New York University Press, 1960.

Shryock, Richard H. *Medicine in America: Historical Essays.* Baltimore: Johns Hopkins University Press, 1966.

Sinai, Nathan, and Odin W. Anderson. *Emergency Maternity and Infant Care.* Ann Arbor, Mich.: University of Michigan, 1948.

Speert, Harold. *The Sloane Hospital Chronicle.* Philadelphia: F. A. Davis Company, 1963.

Spencer, Herbert R. *The History of British Midwifery.* London: John Bale Sons & Danielson, 1927.

Stedman, Thomas L. *Stedman's Medical Dictionary.* 22nd edition. Baltimore: William & Wilkins Company, 1972.

Stevens, Rosemary. *American Medicine and the Public Interest.* New Haven, Conn.: Yale University Press, 1971.

Taylor, Lloyd C., Jr. *The Medical Profession and Social Reform, 1885-1945.* New York: St. Martin's Press, 1974.

Thoms, Herbert. *Chapters in American Obstetrics.* Springfield, Ill.: Charles C.Thomas, 1933.

Thoms, Herbert. *Our Obstetric Heritage: The Story of Safe Childbirth.* Hamden, Conn.: The Shoe String Press, 1960.

Tobey, James A. *Public Health Law.* New York: The Commonwealth Fund, 1939.

Trattner, Walter I. *Crusade for the Children: A History of the National Child Labor Committee and Child Labor Reform in America.* Chicago: Quadrangle Books, 1970.

Wain, Harry. *A History of Preventive Medicine.* Springfield, Ill.: Charles C. Thomas, 1970.

Waite, Frederick C. *History of the New England Female Medical College, 1848-1874.* Boston: Boston University School of Medicine, 1950.

Walsh, Mary Roth. *"Doctors Wanted: No Women Need Apply." Sexual Barriers in the Medical Profession, 1835-1975.* New Haven, Conn.: Yale University Press, 1977.

Wiebe, Robert H. *The Search for Order, 1877-1920.* New York: Hill and Wang, 1967.

Wilcocks, Charles. *Medical Advance, Public Health and Social Evolution.* London: Pergamon Press Ltd., 1965.

Wilkie, K. E., and E. R. Moseley. *Frontier Nurse: Mary Breckinridge.*

New York: Messmer, 1969.

Wilson, Dorothy Clarke. *Lone Woman: The Life of Elizabeth Blackwell.* London: Hodder & Stoughton, 1970.

Woodbury, Robert Morse. *Infant Mortality and Its Causes.* Baltimore: Williams & Wilkins Company, 1926.

Young, James H. *The Medical Messiahs: A Social History of Health Quackery in Twentieth Century America.* Princeton, N.J.: Princeton University Press, 1967.

Young, James H. *The Toadstool Millionaries: A Social History of Patent Medicines in America Before Federal Regulation.* Princeton, N.J.: Princeton University Press, 1961.

Articles

Ackerkneckt, Erwin H. "American Gynecology Around 1850." *Wisconsin Medical Journal,* 51 (1952), 273-274.

"American Women's Hospitals: A Half-Century of Service." *Journal of the American Medical Women's Association,* 22 (August 1967), 548-571.

Anderson, E. G. "History of a Movement: Admission of Women into the Medical Profession." *Fortnightly,* 53 (March 1893), 404-417.

Baer, Joseph L. "A Century of Obstetrics and Gynecology." *Illinois Medical Journal,* 77 (1940), 468-470.

Barker-Benfield, Ben. "The Spermatic Economy: A Nineteenth Century View of Sexuality." *Feminist Studies,* 1 (1970), 45-74.

Baumgartner, Leona. "The American Pattern for Child Health." *Briefs,* 14 (February 1950), 3-7, 14.

Brown, R. Christie. "The History of Midwifery." *Maternity and Child Welfare,* 15 (October-November 1931), 243-245.

Bullough, Vern, and Martha Vought. "Women, Menstruation, and Nineteenth Century Medicine." *Bulletin of the History of Medicine,* 47 (January-February 1973), 66-82.

Burosh, Phyllis. "Physicians' Attitudes Toward Nurse-Midwives." *Nursing Outlook,* 23 (July 1975), 453-456.

Chase, Helen C. "Perinatal and Infant Mortality in the United States and Six West European Countries." *American Journal of Public Health,* 57 (October 1967), 1736-1748.

Christeve, Jackie. "Midwives Busted in Santa Cruz." *Second Wave,* 3 (Summer 1974), 5-10.

Corea, Gena. "Lost Women: Dorothy Reid Mendenhall— 'Childbirth is Not a Disease'." *Ms.,* 2 (April 1974), 98-104.

Dannreuther, Walter. "The American Board of Obstetrics and Gynecology:

Its Origin, Progress and Accomplishments." *American Journal of Obstetrics and Gynecology,* 68 (July 1954), 15-19.

Davis, Dorothy Crane, and Lamar Middleton. "Rebirth of the Midwife." *Today's Health* (February 1968), 28-31, 70-71.

Draeger, Ida J. "Women as Physicians in the United States, 1850-1900." *Bulletin of the History of Medicine,* 16 (1944), 72-81.

Duffy, John. "Masturbation and Clitoridectomy: A Nineteenth Century View." *Journal of the American Medical Association,* 186 (October 1963), 246-248.

Falkner, Frank. "Infant Mortality: An Urgent National Problem." *Children,* 17 (May-June 1970), 83-87.

Ferguson, James H. "Mississippi Midwives." *Journal of the History of Medicine,* 5 (1950), 85-95.

Findley, P. "Midwives' Books." *Medical Life,* 42 (April 1935), 167-186.

Goldberg, Michael. "California Birth Center Busted." *Rough Times,* 4 (March-May 1974), 4.

Goldsmith, Seth B., John W. C. Johnson, and Monroe Lerner. "Obstetricians' Attitudes Toward Nurse-Midwives." *American Journal of Obstetrics and Gynecology,* 111 (September 1971), 111-118.

Goodell, William. "When and Why Were Male Physicians Employed As Accoucheurs?" *American Journal of Obstetrics and the Diseases of Women and Children,* 9 (August 1876), 381-390.

Gordon, J. E. "British Midwives Through the Centuries." *Midwife Health and Visitor,* 3 (1967), 181-187, 237-240, 257-281.

Gordon, Linda. "Voluntary Motherhood: The Beginnings of Feminist Birth Control Ideas in the United States." *Feminist Studies,* 1 (Winter-Spring 1973), 5-22.

Hamilton, M. "Dr. Jesse Bennett-Pioneer Physician." *West Virginia Medical Journal,* 60 (January 1964), 43.

Haydon, M. O. "English Midwives in Three Centuries." *Maternity and Child Welfare,* 3 (1919), 407-409.

Hudson, Robert P. "Abraham Flexner in Perspective: American Medical Education, 1865-1910." *Bulletin of the History of Medicine,* 46 (December 1972), 545-561.

Hunt, Eleanor P., and Alice D. Chenoweth. "Recent Trends in Infant Mortality in the United States." *American Journal of Public Health,* 51 (February 1961), 190-207.

Hurd-Mead, Kate Campbell. "A Study of the Medical Education of Women." *Journal of the American Medical Association,* 116 (January 1941), 339-347.

Jacobson, Paul H. "Hospital Care and the Vanishing Midwife." *Milbank*

Memorial Fund Quarterly, 34 (July 1956), 253-261.

Jensen, Joan M. "Politics and the American Midwife Controversy." *Frontiers*, 1 (Spring 1976), 19-33.

King, Howard D. "The Evolution of the Male Midwife with Some Remarks on the Obstetrical Literature of Other Ages." *American Journal of Obstetrics and the Diseases of Women and Children*, 77 (February 1918), 177-186.

Kobrin, Frances E. "The American Midwife Controversy: A Crisis of Professionalization." *Bulletin of the History of Medicine*, 40 (July-August 1966), 350-363.

Koehler, Lyle. "The Case of the American Jezebels: Anne Hutchinson and Female Agitation During the Years of Antinomian Turmoil, 1636-1640." *William and Mary Quarterly*, 31 (January 1974), 55-78.

Kosmak, George W. "The American Gynecological Society." *American Journal of Surgery*, 51 (1941), 305-306.

Lemons, J. Stanley. "The Sheppard-Towner Act: Progressivism in the 1920's." *Journal of American History*, 55 (March 1969), 776-786.

Leonard, T. A. "History of the Wisconsin Maternal Mortality Study and Survey Committee." *Wisconsin Medical Journal*, 69 (February 1970), 75-78.

Lerner, Gerder. "The Lady and the Mill Girl: Changes in the Status of Women in the Age of Jackson." *Midcontinent American Studies Journal*, 10 (Spring 1969), 5-15.

MacFarlane, Catherine. "Women Physicians and the Medical Societies." *Transactions and Studies of the College of Physicians of Philadelphia*, 26 (1958), 80-83.

Markowitz, Gerald E., and David Karl Rosner. "Doctors in Crisis: A Study of the Use of Medical Education Reform to Establish Modern Professional Elitism in Medicine." *American Quarterly*, 25 (March 1973), 83-107.

Marmol, J. G., A. L. Scriggins, and R. F. Vollman. "History of the Maternal Mortality Study Committees in the United States." *Obstetrics and Gynecology*, 34 (July 1969), 123-138.

Mathews, W. S. "Why Were Physicians Employed as Accoucheurs Instead of Midwives?" *Toledo Medical and Surgical Journal*, 3 (1879), 54-56.

McDaniel, W. B., II. "The Beginning of American Medical Historiography." *Bulletin of the History of Medicine*, 26 (1952), 45-53.

McDaniel, W. G., II. "A View of Nineteenth Century Medical Historiography in the United States of America." *Bulletin of the History of Medicine*, 33 (1959), 415-435.

Mengert, William F. "The Origin of the Male Midwife." *Annals of Medical History*, 4 (September 1932), 453-465.

"Midwives Busted." *Off Our Backs*, 4 (June 1974), 8.

Monroe, Robert F. "Historical Development of Obstetric Education in the South." *Southern Medical Journal*, 52 (1959), 1142-1148.

Moriyama, T. M. "Present Status of the Infant Mortality Problem in the United States." *American Journal of Public Health*, 56 (April 1966), 623-625.

Muckle, Craig W. "The First Five Years: A History of the Beginnings of the American Academy of Obstetrics and Gynecology." *Obstetrics and Gynecology*, 13 (March 1959), 365-374.

Munger, D. B. "Robert Brookings and the Flexner Report." *Journal of the History of Medicine*, 23 (October 1968), 356-371.

Nicodemus, Roy E. "The History of American Obstetrics." *Centaur*, 51 (1945-1946), 25-32.

Noall, Claire. "Mormon Midwives." *Utah Historical Quarterly*, 10 (1942), 84-144.

Pearce, L. "A Century of Medical Education for Women." *Independent Woman*, 29 (April 1950), 104-106.

Rosenberg, Charles E. "Sexuality, Class and Role in Nineteenth-Century America." *American Quarterly*, 25 (May 1973), 131-154.

Rosenberg, Charles E. "Social Class and Medical Care in Nineteenth-Century America: The Rise and Fall of the Dispensary." *Journal of the History of Medicine*, 29 (January 1974), 32-54.

Rosenberg, Charles E., and Carroll S. Rosenberg. "Pietism and the Origins of the American Public Health Movement." *Journal of the History of Medicine*, 23 (1968), 16-35.

Rosenfield, Harold H. "Progress of Obstetrics During the Past Fifty Years." *Rhode Island Medical Journal*, 37 (1954), 498-502.

Rosenkrantz, Barbara Gutman. "Cart Before Horse: Theory, Practice and Professional Image in American Public Health, 1870-1920." *Journal of the History of Medicine*, 29 (January 1974), 55-73.

Schumann, Edward A. "A Century of American Obstetrics and Gynecology." *Quarterly Review of Obstetrics*, 6 (1948), 423-434.

Shapiro, Sam, and I. M. Moriyama. "International Trends in Infant Mortality and Their Implication for the United States." *American Journal of Public Health*, 53 (May 1963), 747-760.

Slemons, Josiah Morris. "Progress in Obstetrics, 1890-1940." *American Journal of Surgery*, 51 (1941), 79-96.

Smith, Daniel Scott. "Family Limitation, Sexual Control and Domestic Feminism." *Feminist Studies*, 1 (Winter-Spring 1973), 40-57.

Smith-Rosenberg, Carroll. "The Hysterical Woman: Sex Roles and Role Conflict in Nineteenth-Century America." *Social Research*, 39 (Winter 1972), 652-678.

Smith-Rosenberg, Carroll. "Puberty to Menopause: The Cycle of Feminity in Nineteenth-Century America." *Feminist Studies*, 1 (Winter-Spring 1973), 58-69.

Smith-Rosenberg, Carroll, and Charles Rosenberg. "The Female Animal: Medical and Biological Views of Women and Her Role in Nineteenth-Century America." *Journal of American History*, 60 (September 1973), 332-356.

Snapper, I. "Midwifery, Past and Present." *Bulletin of the New York Academy of Medicine*, 39 (August 1963), 503-532.

Somer, Carol. "How Women Had Control of Their Bodies and Lost It." *Second Wave*, 2 (1973), 5-10, 28.

Stern, C. A. "Midwives, Male-Midwives, and Nurse-Midwives." *Obstetrics and Gynecology*, 39 (February 1972), 308-311.

Taylor, H. C. "The Making of a Woman's Hospital." *Obstetrics and Gynecology*, 31 (April 1968), 566-574.

Taylor, Howard C., Jr. "Notes on Fifty Years of Progress of Gynecology." *American Journal of Surgery*, 51 (1941), 97-109.

Thomas, T. Gaillard. "A Century of American Medicine, 1776-1876: Obstetrics and Gynecology." *American Journal of the Medical Sciences*, 72 (July 1876), 133-170.

Thoms, Herbert. "The American Obstetric Heritage: An Inspiration in Teaching Obstetrics." *Obstetrics and Gynecology*, 8 (1956), 648-653.

Thoms, Herbert. "Thomas Chalkey James: A Pioneer in the Teaching of Obstetrics in America." *American Journal of Obstetrics and Gynecology*, 29 (February 1935), 289-294.

Tyrone, Curtis. "Certain Aspects of Gynecologic Practice in the Late Nineteenth Century." *American Journal of Surgery*, 84 (1952), 95-106.

Wallace, Helen M., and Hyman Goldstein. "The Status of Infant Mortality in Sweden and the United States." *Journal of Pediatrics*, 87 (December 1975), 995-1000.

Wasserman, Manfred J. "Henry L. Coit and the Certified Milk Movement in the Development of Modern Pediatrics." *Bulletin of the History of Medicine*, 46 (July-August 1972), 359-390.

Weisl, Bernard A. G. "The Nurse-Midwife and the New York City Health Code." *Western Journal of Surgery, Obstetrics and Gynecology*, 71 (November-December 1963), 266-269.

Welter, Barbara. "The Cult of True Womanhood, 1820-1860." *American Quarterly*, 18 (Summer 1966), 151-174.

Unpublished Theses

Buck, Dorothy F. "History of Midwifery." Unpublished Master's thesis,

Teachers College, Columbia University, 1927.

Burrow, James Gordon. "The Political and Social Policies of the AMA, 1901-1941." Unpublished Ph.D. dissertation, University of Illinois, 1956.

Donegan, Janet B. "Midwifery in America, 1760-1860: A Study in Medicine and Morality." Unpublished Ph.D. dissertation, Syracuse University, 1972.

Eickhoff, Harold Walter. "The Organization and Regulation of Medicine in Missouri, 1883-1901." Unpublished Ph.D. dissertation, University of Missouri, 1964.

Fedde, Helen Marie. "A Study of Midwifery with Special Reference to Its Historical Background, Its Present Status, and a Consideration of Its Future in the United States." Unpublished Master's thesis, University of Kentucky, 1950.

Leith, Mary Evelyn. "The Development of Midwife Education in South Carolina, 1919-1946." Unpublished M.A. thesis, Yale University, 1948.

Weiss, Nancy Pottisham. "Save the Children: A History of the Children's Bureau, 1903-1918." Unpublished Ph.D. dissertation, University of California, Los Angeles, 1974.

Miscellaneous

Blake, John B. "Origins of Maternal and Child Health Programs." Mimeographed. Yale University School of Medicine, 1953.

Everett, Houston S. "The History of the American Gynecological Society Prepared for the Celebration of the 100th Anniversary of Its Founding in 1876." Unpublished paper, 1974.

Letter from Carol Fenichel. Reference librarian, Florence A. Moore Library of Medicine, Medical College of Pennsylvania, January 30, 1974.

Letter from Aileen Hogan. Chairwoman, Archives Committee, American College of Nurse-Midwives, July 11, 1974.

Letter from Naomi Patchin. Director, Section on Nursing, American Medical Association, August 12, 1975.

Scholten, Catherine M. " 'On the Importance of the Obstetrick Art': Changing Customs of Childbirth in America, 1760-1825." Forthcoming article in *William and Mary Quarterly*.

Wertz, Dorothy, and Richard Wertz. "Childbirth as Disease." Unpublished paper read at the Second Berkshire Conference on the History of Women, Radcliffe College, Cambridge, Mass., October 26, 1974.

Wertz, Richard, and Dorothy Wertz. "Lying-in, A History of Childbirth in America: Its Technologies and Social Relations." Unpublished manuscript, Boston [1974].

Index

ABOUT THE AUTHOR

Judy Barrett Litoff, assistant professor of history at Bryant College, has specialized in American women's and minority history. Her articles have appeared in *The Historian, Labor History,* and other journals.